HANDBOOK

FOR TOTAL BODY

RE-CONDITIONING

Scientific Weight-Loss

Joint-Ligament-Muscle Conditioning

Aerobics-Balance-Strengthening Exercise

Mental Health-Memory Stimulation

Del Meyer, MD

DISCLOSURE

All Rights Reserved Graphics and video references included in this handbook are part of the public domain and are included herein solely for the purpose of commentary, and/or documentation. Copyrighted material cited herein falls under the Fair Use exemption to U.S. Copyright laws.

The author has referenced many open sources including websites, other authors, as well as decades of his own conference and lecture notes and apologizes if any material appears to be taken from copyrighted sources that have been used over many years in his medical practice and for teaching medical students, nurses, respiratory therapists, and staff with original source no longer available.

Please note: The subject matter in this handbook is controversial and the author largely uses his personal clinical experience in addition to the prevailing scientific evidence assembled over decades of teaching.

For more than 45-years of medical practice he has used the methods recorded in this Handbook with over 10,000 overweight patients, more than half of whom were diabetic and, have benefited from their use. These are now recorded in this handbook for the public.

The medical suggestions herein should NOT be interpreted either as a medical prescription or as coming from a treating source. Always defer to your personal physician's treatment program.

DEDICATION

To My Wife

LINDA ANNETTE

FOR HER HELP

AND

INSIGHT IN TO HEALTHY EATING

APPRECIATION

With special appreciation to

John Loofbourow, MD for help with editing.

In appreciation to Carol Brown, MD

for her initial review and critique.

And last, in appreciation to Jeffrie Rowland

for her assistance in formatting and publishing

this book.

TABLE OF CONTENTS

PART II—PHYSICAL EXERCISE

PART III—THE BRAIN, MEMORY AND COGNITION

PART IV—FOOD LISTS

Self-care is increasingly important.

APHORISMS

Attributing overweight to overeating is hardly more illuminating than ascribing alcoholism to alcohol. —Jean Mayer

All that running and exercise can do for you is make you healthy. —Denny McClain

A vigorous five-mile walk will do more good for an unhappy but otherwise healthy adult than all the medicine and psychology in the world. —Paul Dudley White

Not less than two hours a day should be devoted to exercise. —Thomas Jefferson

Drink a glass of wine after your soup, and you steal a ruble from the doctor. —Russian proverb

The longer I live the less confidence I have in drugs and the greater is my confidence in the regulation and administration of diet and regimen. —John Redman Coxe

We sit at breakfast, we sit on the train on the way to work, we sit at work, we sit at lunch, and we sit all afternoon . . . a hodge-podge of sagging livers, sinking gallbladders, drooping stomachs, compressed intestines and squashed pelvic organs. —John Button, Jr.

We can now prove that large numbers of Americans are dying from sitting on their behinds. —Bruce B. Dan

We are under-exercised as a nation. We look instead of play. We ride instead of walk. Our existence deprives us of the minimum of physical activity essential for healthy living. — John F. Kennedy

FOREWARD

THE DIET—WEIGHT—LOSS CHALLENGE

When we met about twenty years ago, Dr. Meyer was editor of SSV Medicine, the official publication of the three county Sierra Sacramento Valley Medical Societies. He maintains an active blog, and a monthly newsletter. An active physician in Sacramento California for 45 years, he often sees patients with obesity and/or diabetes. As a pulmonologist, specializing in diseases of the lungs, he treats those who are so severely overweight that they cannot breathe well.

Neither obesity nor diabetes can be successfully treated or controlled by anyone except the overweight or diabetic person. No physician, no government, no law or regulation, no family member, friend or anyone else can pull that off because it requires changes in personal behavior, in motivation, and in understanding.

Dr. Meyer's experience led him to shun didactic, 'Doctor's Orders' interactions with his patients, and develop ways to communicate better; to listen and speak.

This Handbook is one result. You, the reader, will note that Dr. Meyer often addresses /you/ directly; you the person rather than the category, diabetic or obese. He shares his own experience with being overweight, and pre-diabetic. Yet he does not talk down; there is enough technical detail here, and enough information to understand the problem and the process of self-care, and self-cure. Dr. Del Meyer offers you the information and the tools so 'You' can overcome.

As Dr. Meyer urges: *Be Well*

John Loofbourow, MD

PREFACE

THE DIET—WEIGHT—LOSS CONUNDRUM

Current data indicates that about one-half to two-thirds of Americans are overweight and suggests that about one-third are obese. After 45 years of medical practice treating more than 40,000 patients in my office, I can affirm the validity of the data concerning the prevalence of obesity and the resultant diabetic, cardiac, and kidney disease. What is frequently not appreciated is the arthritic effect obesity has on our weight bearing joints; the hips, knees, ankles, feet and spine when they are overburdened by excessive weight. This is a serious health problem and frequent cause of disability.

However, there are thousands of diets, weight loss, and exercise programs on the market as can be seen on the bookseller's shelves. Why are they proliferating despite their ineffectiveness? Why is obesity continuing to increase in nearly epidemic proportions? What is missing to make the human body healthy?

We have designed this handbook to cover and unify what is missing in a concise handbook fashion, which is easy to read and to follow. The end-result should be a normal weight, improved cardio-vascular system, improved musculo-skeletal system with a reduction in backache and joint problems and improved mental functioning. Thus, as you follow this handbook, you will enjoy an improvement in both physical (musculo-skeletal, cardiovascular, diabetic) and mental (cognition, memory, well-being) health.

A healthy body is a condition that creates a healthy mind. We have included mental and memory exercises in this handbook for a total body and mind re-conditioning program.

This Scientific Weight Loss, Exercise, Total Body Reconditioning Handbook may be the most important information for your physical and mental health that you have ever read. It is written in a straight forward fashion, so it will be easily understood. It is in Digest Size and soft cover, which makes it easy to carry with you for easy reference as you shop, travel or even dine out. You can download it into your I-pad,

I-pod, or laptop so that you can easily access the references directly from the web with one-click. This makes important information available to you in all aspects of your life and further enlarges your understanding of the totality of your problem.

INTRODUCTION

THE DIET—WEIGHT—EXERCISE—MEMORY DILEMMA

There are many diet and weight loss programs on the market which reflect the high level of public concern and interest in obesity and weight problems. However, the data indicates this weight loss is generally temporary with a rebound to the prior weight or higher.

The CEO of Whole Foods stated that "our nation's fat and sick and we eat terrible diets. We die of heart disease, hypertension, strokes, obesity, and diabetes. These are lifestyle diseases which are largely avoidable or reversible." This was one pattern that he had hoped to change. Changing one's lifestyle and enjoying better and longer health is also one of the higher purposes of this handbook.

In this Handbook, we will provide you with a global unified program for success in achieving your desirable weight and increase your understanding of how foods and specific activities relate to your health and well-being. We will provide advice about diet and exercise for keeping your muscles, tendons, ligaments healthy and joints mobile. We will stress that balance training is increasingly important as we age. We will advise cognitive and memory exercises to preserve your physical and mental health.

EAT WELL

KEEP YOUR WEIGHT NORMAL

ENJOY A LONG, HEALTHY AND SATISFYING LIFE

STAY WELL

CHAPTER 1

PRINCIPLES OF EATING, DIETING AND EXERCISE

For Physical & Mental Health

Health data suggests that maintaining a normal weight and a good aerobic exercise program with muscle strengthening may delay or prevent arthritis, delay or prevent clinical diabetes, improve mental health and well-being, increase productivity and may delay or possibly prevent dementia.

Diets Cannot Cure Obesity (Permanent Weight Loss)

Diets usually cause a temporary drop in weight, which will rebound as soon as you finish the diet. Bob Schwartz (see appendix) has written two books on the subject (Diets Don't Work, and Diets Still Don't Work). He states that after 100 diets he has lost over 2000 pounds but re-gained 2001. I have personally observed this in my practice hundreds of times. When a patient brings up a weight problem, they frequently allege that they don't eat enough to make them obese.

In a restaurant sitting next to a table with three obese women, I was watching their meals being delivered. All were salads on large plates (no salad plates); all had meat, fruit, vegetables, and a large amount of dressing. I visualize these ladies saying, as so many of my patients have done, "Doctor I don't eat much, mostly salads." However, the calories on each plate were easily over a thousand—more than necessary in one meal to maintain their obesity.

Hence, the first goal is to change your eating or dietary habits permanently. Thus, the changes we will recommend must be accepted as a new way of eating or living forever, not just for the few months of a diet.

Diet Pills Cannot Cure Obesity (Permanent Weight Loss)

Diet pills have the same success and failure story. They can normally be given for a short period of time. Most recommendations are to limit them for one to three months if there is no hypertension, strokes or heart disease present. At the end of that reasonably safe period there is frequently rebound weight gain. This weight-gain often exceeds their prior baseline weight, at which point they request another prescription and repeat performance. But I allow this only once every year because of the hazards of these types of drugs. After several treatment periods, charting the course on a graph demonstrates that, in many cases, the increase in weight over the several years is significantly greater than the pretreatment weight. Despite this incontrovertible evidence, patients frequently voice their disbelief. This is also part of the obesity syndrome.

Sugar Substitutes Do Not Help (They Actually Increase Obesity)

A study in the Canadian Medical Association Journal searched the literature for randomly controlled studies involving non-nutritive sweeteners. They found a mere seven trials, with a total of only 1,003 people that evaluated consumption of sugar substitutes for more than six months. They found that sweeteners generally failed to help people lose weight. Most people use sweeteners for controlling or losing weight. However, if this substance was considered a drug instead of a food substance, it would be deemed ineffective based on the best evidence available.

The researchers also looked at 30 observational studies, those that did not involve changing people's diets, but merely cataloging the diet and determining changes over time. They found that people who consumed these sweeteners were more likely to have increases in weight and waistline, and a higher incidence of obesity, hypertension, metabolic syndrome, Type 2 diabetes and cardiovascular events. It is therefore, important to avoid all artificial sweeteners.

Exercise Cannot Cure Obesity (Permanent Weight Loss)

A common rationale given by women is that they have not lost weight because they can't exercise.

A study by the health exercise and rehabilitation group at Bangor University in Wales was done to determine whether exercise causes people to lose weight. They divided their women age 18-34 into two exercise training groups. They recorded the women's body weight, muscle, and fat mass at the start and at the end of the study. They took blood samples to measure appetite hormones and measured their food intake. Results showed that neither lean nor obese women lost weight including the 34 finishers of the four-week exercise program and the 36 finishers of the eight-week exercise program. However, the lean women did gain muscle mass. This confirmed that exercise is not effective in weight control.

It is easier to not eat calories than to burn them off. Unfortunately, food is everywhere, not only in the grocery store, but also in the pharmacies, book stores, gas stations and even hardware stores. And portions are out of control in restaurants.

Most people have no concept of how many calories can be burned with exercise. The slowest eater can eat more calories than an Olympic runner can lose.

For example: if you weigh 175 pounds, you would burn 2 x 175 = 350 / 3.5 = 100 calories per mile. Since there are 3500 calories in 1 lb. of body fat, a 175-pound person needs to walk 35 miles to work off one pound or 350 miles to work off 10 pounds. Most of us would find it impossible to lose weight that way. However, that's a frequent excuse in the consultation room when patients gain weight. "I haven't been able to exercise—that's why I can't lose weight."

That reasoning is totally invalid but keeps surfacing almost daily in a clinical practice. That hurdle must be overcome before you move to being successful in weight loss, which is keeping the weight off.

THE ONLY WAY TO LOSE WEIGHT IS TO EAT LESS BY CUTTING THE PORTIONS OF EACH SERVING YOU PUT ON YOUR PLATE AT MEALTIME, WITH NO SECOND HELPINGS, NO BETWEEN MEAL OR BEDTIME SNACKS OR SODAS. REMEMBER, WHETHER SODAS ARE SWEETENED WITH SUGAR OR ARTIFICAL SWEETENERS, THEY INHIBIT YOUR WEIGHT-LOSS PROGRAM AND INCREASE YOUR RISKS FOR GETTING

CARDIOVASCULAR DISEASE AND STROKES. REPLACE THOSE SNACKS WITH A HALF GLASS OF WATER OR CHEW ON A CARROT OR PIECE OF CELERY INSTEAD.

REMEMBER ALSO THAT CARBOHYDRATES CAN COME IN MANY FORMS BESIDES SIMPLE SUGARS: SUCH AS STARCHY VEGETABLES, GRAINS, INCLUDING RICE, BREAD, AND PASTA. WHOLE GRAIN FOODS MAY BE HEALTHIER, BUT NOT WITH REGARD TO CALORIES.

Men following these simple rules of no second helpings or between meals or bedtime snacks will lose approximately 50 pounds in the first year with no other change in their diets.

Women following these simple rules of no second helpings or between meals or bedtime snacks will lose approximately 25 pounds in the first year with no other change in their diets.

Hence, you may not even need a doctor or see a dietician if you do this first. Just think about the health care costs you then will save.

Do a Trial Run

If you can do this for 8 weeks, and lose 8 pounds, then you will be successful in returning to a normal weight with improved physical and mental health and well-being.

IF YOU CANNOT PASS THIS TRIAL RUN, consider giving this book to someone interested in losing their excess weight and returning their bodies to health and healing.

* * * * *

Patient Anecdote

Explaining diets, weight loss, and eating less may seem obvious to most health-care professionals. But just as Martin Luther stated that children are sometimes the best teachers for parents, so too, our patients can be good teachers for us. That is as true in 2017 as it was in 1517.

After what seems like an obvious explanation by the physician to the patient, sometimes it's only after the patient response that we fully appreciate the level of understanding they may have. After explaining the concept of taking fewer and smaller helpings of all the food we put on our plate, one man stated, "So that's how you can eat less. I've never understood before how one can eat less."

CHAPTER 2

WHAT IS A NORMAL WEIGHT?

The levels of overweight and obesity in countries like the USA or UK are much higher than in countries such as The Netherlands. Therefore, a Dutch person may aim for a lower ideal weight than an American if all he did was to compare himself to other people there. We will use the charts designed for the USA that define the weight, which is relative to our height. This correlation defines our Body Mass Index.

There are several height/weight charts readily available. We have referenced the National Institute of Health and their standard "body mass index" (BMI) charts. This is not a textbook but a Guide-Book, so we will keep this our basic goal and keep it simple.

The Weight and Height guide chart uses the National Institute of Health's body mass index tables to determine how much your healthy weight should be for your height. Click to review. The NIH and CDC (Center for Disease Control) have calculators in which you enter your height and weight to calculate your BMI.

Is the BMI chart for everyone?

BMI is a very simple measurement, which does not take in to account the person's waist, chest or hip measurements. As an extreme example of this, an Olympic 100m sprint champion is likely to have a BMI higher than a couch potato of the same height. The couch potato may have a big belly, not much muscle and a lot of fat on his hips, upper thighs, and on other parts of his body. While the athlete will have a smaller waist, much less body fat, but more muscle mass and will most likely enjoy better health. Using a pure BMI criterion, might make the couch potato seem as healthy as the athlete.

BMI does not take bone density (bone mass) into account. A person with severe osteoporosis (very low bone density) may have a lower BMI than somebody else of the same height who is healthy, but the person with osteoporosis may have a larger waist, more body fat and weak bones.

The BMI chart is for general use for adults and is the one we will utilize. Children have their own chart with a different set of normal variations which also includes an age variation as well as percentile bands. A percentile of 50 indicates that half of the children are over, and half are under your weight. It means that if a child is in the 50th percentile that child is average, or, normal. If in the 90th percentile the child is overweight or, abnormal by comparison to other children of the same age and height.

Charts for Children

As of 2015, an ideal height and weight chart for children can be found at Merck Manual and the Center for Disease Control and Prevention. The Merck Manuals use charts with age on the x-axis, and height, or weight, on the y-axis. All charts contain bands representing different percentiles which indicate your place with your peers.

Normal weight varies greatly from infancy, through childhood and adolescence. Normal weight also varies greatly between men and women. There are many studies and charts that have been devised over the years. The height and weight charts offered by the Centers for Disease Control and Prevention list heights, weights and the percentile of people at or above that measurement for every age, up to 20 years old. People use these charts to track growth and compare height and weight with national averages. Each chart has lines for height and weight corresponding to the 5th, 25th, 50th, 75th and 95th percentiles at every age from 2 to 20. The CDC offers charts for boys and girls and has separate charts for children from birth until 36 months. How a chart works varies depending on the chart. Multiple types of height and weight charts are available. The 90th percentile means the individual is taller or heavier than 90 percent of children of the same age.

Charts for Women

Women have a different form of fat distribution. This also includes variations for their individual frame. Therefore, separate charts are frequently used for women.

One place to find a height and weight chart for women is on Rush University Medical Center's official website, www.Rush.edu. The charts from Rush University Medical center stand out as one that is generally recognized as valid.

Charts for women frequently also include variations for their frame. These are important after achieving a normal BMI on the standard charts.

What is your ideal body weight?

This handbook will focus its discussion on age 17/18 or at the point of high school graduation which some experts label as the ideal body weight. Others define your ideal body weight as your weight at age 21/22 when you finish college or reach adulthood, while others use age 24/25 when you enter your life work or profession.

The National Health Service has a height and weight chart for adults that uses color shades to indicate whether certain height and weight combinations are underweight, healthy, overweight, obese or very obese. This chart is closely related to body mass index, a number rating that indicates a person's health according to height and weight. Body mass index and height and weight charts are sometimes inaccurate, as they can classify a healthy person as overweight if he has a large amount of muscle mass.

Our first goal and the purpose of this handbook is to attain a normal weight for our height. We will define as a normal BMI, for which we will use the chart reproduced in Chapter 4.

Remember

In general, it is best to avoid starchy foods such as potatoes, rice, breads, and sweetened foods, like cereal soaked in sugar, donuts, sweet rolls, sweet desserts, candy, sodas, diet sodas or artificial sweeteners.

Birthdays and Holidays are excluded, but only in very small amounts.

CHAPTER 3

WHAT IS OBESITY?

Weighing more than can be justified by your height...

Weight should be proportional to one's height. A 7' man weighing 275 pounds is not overweight while a 5'2" female weighing 175 pounds is overweight. This ratio indicates the Body Mass Index, which can be determined by one's own measurements using a complicated formula. For practical purposes, however, we will use the BMI charts that have been pre-calculated. When weight is proportional to one's height, obesity is not present. This proportionality has been codified in tables for easy reference. If weight is larger than the normal relationship of weight to height, then one is obese. If the weight is less than the normal relationship of weight to height, then one is underweight.

How Did You Become Overweight?

By eating more than you need for your daily body activity and maintenance of baseline weight, which is approximately ten calories per pound.

The first goal for two-thirds of the population is weight assessment and control. This allows most of us to begin traveling the road to a healthy body without the assessment of a physician, nurse or dietician.

The food we eat provides calories. Weight gain or loss is the difference between the calories we eat and the calories we use. Every excess of 500 calories per day or 3500 calories per week that we eat beyond what we expend in our daily work equals one pound of weight gain per week. Every decrease of 500 calories per day or 3500 calories per week in our diet below what we expend in our daily activities equals one pound of weight loss per week. 3500 Calories = one pound.

Thus eating 500 calories more than are required for your energy/work load and to maintain your weight every day is an excess of 3500 calories per week or one-pound of weight gain per week.

Eating 500 fewer calories than are required for your energy/work load and to maintain your weight every day will result in a one-pound weight loss per week.

Calories, a basic unit of energy, vary with the type of food.

This energy measurement of food essentially follows the second law of thermodynamics. The current debate over some theoretical issues is not clinically significant or relevant in human dietary management. Thus, the general definition of a calorie is as follows:

- ☐ 1a: the amount of heat required at a pressure of one atmosphere to raise the temperature of one gram of water one degree Celsius—abbreviation cal —also called gram calorie or small calorie- c.
- ☐ 1b: A kilo-calorie is the amount of heat required to raise the temperature of one kilogram of water one degree Celsius: 1000 gram calories—abbreviation C —also called the large calorie
- ☐ 2a: In diets we use a unit equivalent to the large calorie – C expressing heat-producing or energy-producing value in food when oxidized in the body
- ☐ 2b: Thus, a food value of one kilocalorie, C, is equal to an amount of food having an energy-producing value of one large calorie.

500 calories per day or 3500 calories per week will equal one pound of weight. Every pound of weight requires 10 C per day to maintain it.

That means a 150-pound person will require approximately a 1500 Calorie diet to maintain a normal 150-pound person.

And a 200-pound person will require 2000 Calories to maintain a normal 200-pound person.

Therefore, one must be careful when reading the food values on purchased food.

If you eat the amount recommended for a 2000 calorie chart, you will eventually equilibrate at 200 pounds, even if your current weight is 150-pounds. Or conversely, if you weigh 200 pounds and follow the 1500 calorie chart, you will eventually equilibrate at 150 pounds.

25

Calories and weight is a simple equation even if difficult to solve.

Carbohydrates produce 4 Calories per gram when digested, metabolized and oxidized. Thus, one ounce or 30 grams of Carbohydrate will equal 120 Calories and 120-grams, or 4 ounces will provide 480 Calories.

Proteins produce 4 Calories per gram when digested, metabolized and oxidized. Thus, one ounce or 30 grams of Protein will equal 120 Calories and 120-grams or four-ounces of meat, (beef, chicken, turkey, or pork) will provide 480 Calories.

Alcohol produces 7 calories per gram. A shot (1.5 oz) of 80 proof liquor (40 percent alcohol), or a 5 oz glass of 12% wine, or a 12 oz glass of 5% beer all have essentially the same amount of alcohol (0.6 oz or 18 gm or 125 Calories). (There will be a slight variation since liquor, wine, and beer now come with various concentrations of alcohol.) These calculations are only valid for straight or "neat" drinkers. If you use mix, the calories may be several times higher, because of the sugary mix.

Fats produce 9 Calories per gram when digested, metabolized and oxidized. Thus 10 gm is 90 Calories and 30 gm (or one ounce) is 270 Calories and four-ounces or 120 gm is about a thousand Calories.

* * * * *

Patient Anecdote

We had one patient who frequently brought a gift of marbled steaks, which we had to severely trim. As a butcher, he considered lean beef to be inferior. He couldn't understand that fat was related to coronary disease. Despite our caution, the patient either couldn't understand our concerns or simply ignored them. He died in his fifties of a coronary thrombosis. His wife tried unsuccessfully for ten years to make it a military service-connected condition, until her daughter convinced her to quit.

CHAPTER 4

THE BODY MASS INDEX (BMI) TABLE

Body mass index, or BMI, reflects the amount of body fat for adult men and women based on their height and weight, the Centers for Disease Control and Prevention explains. It is a general screening tool for health and obesity.

Testing for BMI is cheap and easy for clinicians, as it requires only the height and weight of an individual. The measurement involves dividing a person's weight in kilograms by the square of height in meters.

People who have a high BMI are at risk for many diseases and health conditions, such as hypertension, high cholesterol, type 2 diabetes, heart disease and strokes. Early diagnosis and correction helps put the person back on track to a healthy life.

BMI does not measure body fat directly. To determine if a high BMI has resulted in an increased health risk, a health care provider may need to perform further tests to screen for certain health problems.

In this handbook we will be using the BMI from the charts provided herein, which are adequate for our purpose of returning to a normal weight. After meeting this initial goal and maintaining it, your physician may require a more sophisticated and personal dietary plan tuned to your specific medical requirements.

BMI Chart and Weight

The following BMI Chart displays what category each BMI falls into: whether underweight, normal, or another category of obesity. The formula used to calculate BMI can be found below as well as here: BMI Formula.

WEIGHT	lbs	90	100	110	120	130	140	150	160	170	180	190	200	210	220	230	240	250	260	270	280	290
	kgs	41	45	50	54	59	64	68	73	77	82	86	91	95	100	104	109	113	118	122	127	132
HEIGHT ft/in	cm	Underweight				Healthy				Overweight				Obese					Extremely Obese			
4'8"	142.2	20	22	25	27	29	31	34	36	38												
4'9"	144.7	19	22	24	26	28	30	32	35	37	39											
4'10"	147.3	19	21	23	25	27	29	31	33	36	38											
4'11"	149.8	18	20	22	24	26	28	30	32	34	36	38										
4'12"	152.4	18	20	21	23	25	27	29	31	33	35	37	39									
5'1"	154.9	17	19	21	23	25	26	28	30	32	34	36	38									
5'2"	157.4	16	18	20	22	24	26	27	29	31	33	35	37	38								
5'3"	160.0	16	18	19	21	23	25	27	28	30	32	34	35	37	39							
5'4"	162.5	15	17	19	21	22	24	26	27	29	31	33	34	36	38	39						
5'5"	165.1	15	17	18	20	22	23	25	27	28	30	32	33	35	37	38						
5'6"	167.6	15	16	18	19	21	23	24	26	27	29	31	32	34	36	37	39					
5'7"	170.1	14	16	17	19	20	22	24	25	27	28	30	31	33	34	36	38	39				
5'8"	172.7	14	15	17	18	20	21	23	24	26	27	29	30	32	33	35	37	38				
5'9"	175.2	13	15	16	18	19	21	22	24	25	27	28	30	31	33	34	35	37	38			
5'10"	177.8	13	14	16	17	19	20	22	23	24	26	27	29	30	32	33	34	36	37	39		
5'11"	180.3	13	14	15	17	18	20	21	22	24	25	27	28	29	31	32	33	35	36	38	39	
5'12"	182.8	12	14	15	16	18	19	20	22	23	24	26	27	28	30	31	33	34	35	37	38	39
6'1"	185.4	12	13	15	16	17	18	20	21	22	24	25	26	28	29	30	32	33	34	36	37	38
6'2"	187.9	12	13	14	15	17	18	19	21	22	23	24	26	27	28	30	31	32	33	35	36	37
6'3"	190.5	11	13	14	15	16	18	19	20	21	23	24	25	26	28	29	30	31	33	34	35	36
6'4"	193.0	11	12	13	15	16	17	18	19	21	22	23	24	26	27	28	29	30	32	33	34	35
6'5"	195.5	11	12	13	14	15	17	18	19	20	21	23	24	25	26	27	28	30	31	32	33	34
6'6"	198.1	10	12	13	14	15	16	17	18	20	21	22	23	24	25	27	28	29	30	31	32	34
6'7"	200.6	10	11	12	14	15	16	17	18	19	20	21	23	24	25	26	27	28	29	30	32	33
6'8"	203.2	10	11	12	13	14	15	16	18	19	20	21	22	23	24	25	26	27	29	30	31	32
6'9"	205.7	10	11	12	13	14	15	16	17	18	19	20	21	23	24	25	26	27	28	29	30	31
6'10"	208.2	9	10	12	13	14	15	16	17	18	19	20	21	22	23	24	25	26	27	28	29	30
6'11"	210.8	9	10	11	12	13	14	15	16	17	18	19	20	21	22	23	24	25	26	27	28	29	30

How to read the BMI Chart

To view where your BMI lies in this chart, first find your weight on the top horizontal axis and then follow the BMI numbers all the way down until the height on the left axis corresponds to your height. The category that your body mass index (BMI) lies under is shaded in the corresponding color which is shown in the legend above as well as listed below:

- Blue: The category is Underweight and corresponds to a BMI of less than 20.
- Green: The category is Normal Weight and corresponds to a BMI between 20 and 25.
- Yellow: The category is Overweight and corresponds to a BMI of 25 to 30.
- Orange: The category is Obese and corresponds to a BMI between 30 and 40.
- Some authors define Class One obesity as a BMI of between 30 and 35.

- The same authors then define Class Two obesity as a BMI of between 35 and 40.
- Red: The category is Extremely Obese and corresponds to a BMI of 40 or higher. This may then be classified as Stage Three obesity.
- Some authors label a BMI of over 50 as being Morbidly Obese.

What is your BMI? Is it normal or obese?

- What is your current weight: _____ Pounds
- What is your current height? _____ Feet _____ Inches
- Read your current BMI from the Table: _____

What is your weight category?

What is my weight category from the chart above?
- Normal: 20-25 _____
- Overweight: 25-30 _____
- Stage One Obesity: 30-35 _____
- Stage Two Obesity: 35-40 _____
- Stage Three Obesity: 40-50 _____
- Morbid Obesity: < 50 _____

Determine your initial goal:

Find your present BMI from the table.
- Move your finger to the left along your height line to the GREEN ZONE
- Then move upward to the weight line.
- Use any weight number that corresponds to the green height number that you would like to set as your first goal. Subtract that from your present weight _____
- Your total weight loss to reach your personal goal of a BMI of 20-25 _____
- Or if obese, go for BMI of 25-30 in the mildly overweight zone: _____
- Enter the number of months you wish to take to reach your ideal weight: _____
- Enter a number such as 3 months, 6 months, 9 months, or 12 months: _____

- Remember: every 3500 calories per week or 500 calories reduction per day will equal one pound of weight loss per week.
- Weigh yourself daily and record your weight. (Use a calendar, graph, or your iPod)
- Or weigh at least every week if you don't have a bathroom scale and record the weight each time. (Use a calendar, graph or iPod)
- You need to invest in a bathroom scale if you're serious about a healthy weight.

DO NOT VIOLATE THE PRINCIPLES OF EATING, LISTED IN CHAPTER 1.

THE ONLY WAY TO LOSE WEIGHT IS TO EAT LESS; NO SECONDS AND NO SNACKS.

LIMIT CAKE, PIE, DESSERTS, AND ICE CREAM TO BIRTHDAYS AND HOLIDAYS WITH FAMILY AND FRIENDS AND EVEN THEN, IN VERY SMALL AMOUNTS.

CHAPTER 5

HOW WEIGHT GAIN CAN SLIP UP ON YOU

There is a lot of misunderstanding about diets and weight gain. For instance, a retired bank executive couldn't understand his 18-pound weight gain over the previous 12 weeks. He had obtained dietary counseling and was told that fruit was a free addition. But fruit, although healthy, contains calories. We determined that the fruit he ate contained 750 calories per day. This would calculate to a one and one-half pound weight gain per week for 12 weeks or the 18-pound gain that he experienced.

Some people wonder how they are supposed to know what to eat if their doctor doesn't tell them. So, I gave my 2000 calorie regimen to one of my sleep apneic patients whose weight has always been above 350 pounds. Her initial response was that she didn't come close to eating that much, which is a typical response. By standard criteria we discussed previously I knew she was eating approximately 3500 calories, per day. However, within one month, my scale weighed her at 344 pounds. Six pounds of weight loss in one month on 2000 calories does indicate that she had been eating more than 2000 calories; So, surprise, 2000 calories were a weight reduction diet for her.

Your Weight Gain Inventory

Puberty: What was your weight and height at puberty or age 12-14, or when you completed primary school?

Weight: _____ lbs. Height: _____ in.

BMI: _____ (from the BMI table)

The first indication of weight gain can be seen by pubescence or the early teenage years. If weight is above normal, that is the time to begin to curb your caloric intake.

If you're eating more than your fellow classmates and you think you're a little chubby, begin to note where you should cut the calories. Eating smaller portions and omitting second

31

portions may be all that you need to lose weight. By the end of the year, you should see if you've been successful.

What was your weight at age 17 or 18 or when you completed high school?

Weight: _____ lbs. Height: _____ in.

BMI: _____ (from the BMI table)

Many nutritionists use this weight as your ideal body weight. If you're overweight at this age, now is the time to curb your appetite and your intake. Again, just making your portions smaller and omitting seconds may bring you back into the normal levels. Changing the weight gain trajectory just a little now may bring you back into the normal weight curve.

What was your weight at age 24 or 25 when you completed college or entered your career or married?

Weight: _____ lbs. Height: _____ in.

BMI: _____ (from the BMI table)

At this stage of your maturity, things generally settle down. There is normally only a modest weight gain at this point in one's life. However, if you are overweight use this as the point to return to as your ideal goal. Then look for a reasonable endpoint for any further weight reduction.

That means smaller portions, no second helpings, and no snacking to point you to your goal even before you can make the appointment to check with your physician or nutritionist.

What should be your weight loss goal?

With your physician or dietitian, determine what should be your appropriate weight loss goal.

Normally this would be the BMI for your present age and height. If you're more than 50 lbs. over, you may want to split this into a two-year effort.

Your physician may determine that your best weight loss goal should be some other number than a goal you may have set for yourself. This could be determined by your BMI at age 17-18 or at age 24-25. If you have medical problems such as diabetes (you know you need to avoid carbohydrates and sweets) or hypertension (you already know to avoid salt) or hyperlipidemia (you already know to avoid saturated fats such as beef and dairy products), your physician may suggest some other goal with other dietary conditions.

My doctor used my weight at age 34 when I had completed my professional training and my post-doctoral work. I still have 10 pounds to lose. However, I have a strong resistance to that from my wife who measures things from the look of my face, to make sure it is not gaunt, and the color is good. Since she is the most important person in the world to me, I may never lose that final 10 pounds my doctor set as my goal.

How to Achieve Normal Weight

Step I: Reduce the number of helpings

If you usually place 5 helpings on your plate, try to reduce it to four, if you normally place 4 helpings on your place, try to reduce it to three.

Step II: Reduce the size of helpings – portion control.

If you usually have 6 or 8 oz. of meat, try for 4 oz. If you usually have 3 small potatoes, try for 2. If you flood your salad with dressing, try to cut that in half. You could even try having your dressing on-the-side and dipping the fork tines into the dressing before each bite of salad. By doing this, you use less dressing, but still have a taste with each bite.

Step III: No second helpings. Just say, "No, thank you."

Step IV: No between meal snacks.

Don't look at the snack. Just say "No thank you" and then look or walk away.

Step V: No bedtime snacks.

Walk away from the temptation or go to bed.

CHAPTER 6

THE DIET INDUSTRY

Obesity is Not a New Disease

Obesity and the desire to conquer it are nothing new. In the 1830s, Presbyterian minister Sylvester Graham ran health retreats to help people lose weight on a diet devoid of meat but heavy on his namesake graham crackers, according to CNN.com. The cigarette industry tried to get in on the diet act in the mid-20th century, promoting its products as a way to lose a few pounds.

For years, Americans cycled through one brand-name diet after another, each promising a sure method to lose weight. Along the way, Jenny Craig, Weight Watchers and Lean Cuisine made fortunes off their low-calorie, low-fat diet programs and products.

But it seems those days may be over. According to industry analysts and nutritionists, "Dieting is not a fashionable word these days," says Susan Roberts, a professor of nutrition and psychiatry at Tufts University. "[Consumers] equate the word diet with deprivation, and they know deprivation doesn't work."

"Consumers are not dieting in the traditional sense anymore – being on programs or buying foods specific to programs," says Marissa Gilbert, an analyst from Mintel who worked on the report. From summer 2014 to summer 2015, Lean Cuisine's frozen meal sales dropped from around $700 million to about $600 million, or about 15 percent. Weight Watchers, Medi-Fast and Jenny Craig have also seen revenues wither over the past few years. Sales of diet pills have dropped 20 percent in the last year, according to the Mintel report.

The Diet Industry Keeps Growing

Despite the fact that diet foods may be tanking, the diet industry is still flourishing. At one bookstore, I counted 107 different diet books. At another there were over 200 titles. At a third, there were six bookcases with five 36-inch shelves (180 inches of shelving x 6 cases), which equals more than a thousand inches of shelving devoted to diet and nutrition. But is there really any new information? It is interesting that as this deluge of diet books is filling up the shelves, other books containing medical dietary information are on sale at 10 percent of their initial listing. Why is the industry flourishing and the results tanking?

Of all the books that cross my desk each month asking for a review, there is at least one or two about dieting. I have reviewed many of these over my 45 years of medical practice and posted many of them on my website. http://delmeyer.net/physicianpatient-bookshelf/

I have also noted that since my current activity in evaluating diets, my inbox has 60 or more daily promotional email notes concerning diet, weight loss, nutrition, surgical procedures and various exercise programs; many promise a three-day, one week, or one-month result. Some say no exercise is required. Some even project the number of pounds to be lost in the projected days (without exercise) without any rational basis for the statements rendered. (Isn't it interesting how the industry found out about my private efforts in writing this handbook before it is even published? And I have not been involved in any social media for four years.) Why has personal information become so ubiquitous?

I was interested in clock-watching one hour of television. There were more than 12 advertisements concerning food, especially desserts. With digital programing, one may see 3 to 10 second insertions in another commercial. That's an average food related ad every five minutes! Diabetics are known to have a "sweet tooth" and once they see a dessert, they must have it. (I must taste it.)

When I eat in the Medical Staff Lounge at my hospital, there is a salad bar, a dessert bar, and a hot food presentation. I fix my salad at the cold salad bar but turn my head away from the dessert bar—I talk to my colleagues, who may already be at the nearby tables, or distract myself in some fashion away from the sweets, until I get to the main menu of hot items of meat, fish and vegetables. I know temptation is frequently overwhelming, so I make sure I never look over the sweets. If I look, I know I've reached the point of not being able to decline.

When a journalist from a local magazine did an interview in my office on diets, I thought I presented the above rather clearly—don't even look at the dessert menu. When the magazine arrived in my office, the editor stated that "I have to see the desserts menu" missing my entire point of NOT looking at the dessert or the dessert menu. Obviously, she could not fathom looking over the dessert menu as a temptation to avoid.

I've also noted when eating out with friends, the women state they can't have desserts but then insist on seeing the dessert menu. They ask the men for their choice and we usually decline. Then the women order large sweet desserts and eat about one-third or less and then give it to their spouses. So, sometimes it is hard to avoid desserts even when one avoids the dessert menu.

There are many diet books written by celebrities. These authors may be without any nutrition credentials. However, some of these books are quite informative and meet a need, which may be attributed to a co-author with nutritional credentials who is working in the field. This may include an MS in nutrition or a PhD, or M.D who work and have clinical experience. The latter group, however, may not always be as knowledgeable as the public assumes.

The Pritikin Diet Reversed Coronary Disease in Mr. Pritikin

Some, such as Nathan Pritikin, an engineer who had a life-threatening coronary problem and had been recommended for a coronary artery procedure, declined the surgery and decided to cure himself medically. As a result, he reversed his coronary artery disease becoming a nutrition expert by his own serious study and experience. He developed the Pritikin Center which was very successful. Unfortunately, his leukemia caught up with him in the end. However, his autopsy revealed completely normal coronary arteries. One pathologist observed they were as soft as a newborn baby's arteries.

Diets Still Don't Work

Searching the archives in my study, I found an audiotape from 1985 titled, Diets Don't Work by Bob Schwartz (Breakthru Publishing, $9.95). I then obtained his book as well as a second book, Diets still Don't Work. Schwartz owned 16 health clubs at age 30 when he put on an extra 40 pounds. Ten years and 100 diets later, he had lost more than 2,000 pounds – and gained back 2,001 pounds. He decided it made as much sense to study fat people if you're interested in losing weight as to study poor people if you're interested in making money. So, he began to study the club members who seemed to stay thin.

He came up with several tips. Eat only when you are hungry. Stop eating when you're no longer hungry – rather than when you're full. Don't dine out more than once or twice a week; restaurant food is usually higher in fat, calories and salt. Avoid sweet rolls, donuts, pastries, most desserts and candy.

He points out that people exercise for the wrong reason–to utilize or burn calories to lose weight. Exercise is important in the overall health program, but it takes 30 minutes of aerobic exercise to work off 12 corn chips. Or walk a mile to work off 100 calories. Very few of us exercise enough to even work off one dessert—three miles for a 300-calorie dessert. The slowest eater can eat more calories than the most vigorous exerciser can lose.

The Diet Industry Continues to Grow

According to Schwartz, the diet industry was spending $33 billion in 1985 to convince us that the only way to lose weight is through dieting. He cited a statistic that 190 people out of 200 do not meet their first goal in the weight reduction programs. Of the 10 that do, nine regain the weight lost and only one of the 200 maintains the weight loss. This, he felt, proved that diets don't work. The diet industry countered that all 200 had lost weight, 10 reached the first goal and, therefore, diets do work – it's the people that don't. The more recent data from 2010 indicates the diet industry is up to $40 billion in the United States and $55 billion globally.

The Industry Continues to grow and related healthcare costs related to Obesity even more. To review extensive statistics: WalletHub recently released a study on obesity rates in the U.S.

Here are some key findings from the report:
- More than 7 in 10 U.S. adults aged 20 and older are either overweight or obese.
- This year, Americans are expected to spend $68 billion on weight-loss programs.
- The U.S. spends nearly $200 billion in annual health care costs related to obesity.
- 81.5 million Americans aged 6 and older were completely inactive in 2016.
- Mississippi had the highest rate of obesity and overweight.
- Colorado had the lowest rate of obesity and overweight.

Diet Analysis—How much do you Eat?

Carrie Latt Wiatt, MS, in her book (Portion Savvy, Pocket Books) discusses interviews with her celebrity clientele. She does a diet inventory and seldom has to get beyond breakfast to convince her clients that they are eating up to 1000 calories beyond what is necessary to support their weight. An extra 1000 calories per day would equal 7000 calories a week or a two-pound weight gain per week. Hence, in a 52-week year, one would gain over 100 pounds, which was exactly why her client came in having gained that much in one year. The client quickly understood why she gained so much weight and immediately cut the portions of all her food. She had overlooked that even healthy food has calories. Over eating is a very common but poorly understood problem in obesity.

I've had many patients who join various programs, lose an expected amount of weight and then rewarded themselves with a "decadent dessert," which, of course, perpetuates the industry and keeps half of Americans overweight.

Are Diets Counter-Productive?

This idea was highlighted in a book which appeared about the same time, "Does Dieting Make You Fat?" by Geoffrey Cannon and Hetty Einzig (Simon & Schuster, 1985, $15.95). It pointed out that, all too often, dieting contributes to the very condition it is meant to cure. Many people think of diets as a temporary unpleasant experience before they can return to their previous eating habits. Thus, the long-term effect of dieting is nil in most cases and in some it is counter-productive.

More recently, patients turn to the web for diet information. Email come in daily offering free diets, how to lose weight while eating everything you want, or even how to get paid for dieting and losing weight.

Web-based Nutritional Websites are only partially effective.

Brown University researchers found that people who had regular online interaction with a dietitian lost more weight than those who simply down loaded a weight-loss plan to follow themselves.

The Tufts University Health & Nutrition Letter, in a recent supplement, rated the weight-loss web sites. Of the free sites, Tufts chooses the easy-to-use "Shape Up America" site, www.shapeup.org, operated by former Surgeon General C. Everett Koop, MD, who also operates the fee-based "Shape Up and Drop 10" site. However, of the fee sites, Tufts recommends the "eDiets" site, www.ediets.com.

CHAPTER 7

AUTHOR'S PERSONAL EXPERIENCE WITH WEIGHT LOSS

When I had my annual physical examination a number of years ago, my doctor told me that I should lose 30 pounds if I wanted to live a longer healthier life. My weight was 220 pounds; my mass body index was 30, bordering Class One obesity.

My mother had diabetes. I, therefore, was at risk for developing diabetes. A paternal cousin had diabetes. With diabetic genes on both sides of my family, the risks were increased.

At standard weight maintenance of 10 calories per pound, I calculated that my diet was about 2200 calories per day. With one pound of body fat equal to 3500 calories, I knew if I removed a fourth of the food from my plate, that should be about 500 calories a day less or 3500 calories less per week which would be equivalent to losing one pound per week. Losing weight is simply a mathematical equation, even if it isn't easy to use.

My doctor didn't have to point out that diabetes destroys our body attacking our retinae, kidneys and peripheral nerves. These result in becoming blind, developing neuropathy, peripheral vascular disease progressing to gangrene with possible amputations, or kidney failure, (the common causes of death from diabetes), which I had observed first hand for more than 40 years of practice. It was a simple conclusion that I better lose 30 pounds before it was too late.

He didn't send me to a dietitian because he knew that I understood how calories and weight were in a direct relationship. He put me on Metformin to try to prevent diabetes, but I was on my own to lose the weight and re-condition my body.

I decided I would make rough estimates by decreasing the portions of my meals. I normally had four portions of the various items and then I eliminated one. So, for instance, when

I went through the Hospital Cafeteria line, I only placed three items on my plate instead of the usual four and made these three portions smaller than usual. I would choose a small salad, and then progress to the hot food meat and vegetable area. I would turn my head away from the dessert area as I walked by to avoid any temptations. At the hot food area, I would take one vegetable instead of two and take a 4 oz. piece of fish, turkey, or chicken. I expected to lose one pound per week.

In two months or eight weeks, I expected to lose 8 pounds. However, I lost 12 pounds. Therefore, I over-estimated how many calories I removed from my plate each day. So that would calculate to 750 calories that I removed each day or 5250 calories in a week instead of the 3500 calories necessary to lose one pound per week. The 1750 calories above 3500 would equal an additional one-half pound per week of excess weight loss. And I was still eating the same food and I was never hungry.

After four months or 16 weeks I expected to lose 16 pounds. However, I lost 20 pounds. Hence, I still overestimated the 500 calories per day required to be removed from my plate each day. It calculated to 625 calories I removed per day. (It was 4375 calories instead of the 3500 calories necessary to lose one pound per week.) I was still eating the same food I was used to eating and was not hungry or having any cravings.

After six months or 24 weeks, I expected to lose 24 pounds. However, I lost the entire 30 pounds my doctor recommended. I returned to my ideal body weight of 190 pounds or a normal BMI of 24 within six months.

It was important that I continue with the small portions, so I wouldn't regain the weight. The reason most diets fail is that patients can't wait to complete the diet and get off it so that they can eat as much of the food they prefer which then restores the prior weight. Since I was always eating the food I preferred, rather than being told what to eat, I had no craving for foods that I was used to eating.

Now this points out another reason for failure. When people are given a new diet with unfamiliar foods, there is almost a zero percentage of success. In this guide book, our first goal is to restore a normal weight. The specialized diets, if necessary for medical problems, would be a subsequent step.

In my case, it was appropriate that I continue with my usual diet in smaller and fewer portions. Thus, I never experienced cravings since I was still eating foods I enjoy.

Some ten years earlier, and because of my hyperlipidemia, my doctor placed me on Statins. After nine months I developed severe cramps in my legs, a known side effect of statins. He then tried a different type of cholesterol medication. I had the same side effect within one week. So, I was on my own to eliminate fatty foods from my diet. My cholesterol was 220 before the statins and 200 after the statins. My triglycerides were 180 mg%.

With a family history of cardiovascular disease, it was imperative that I reduce my cholesterol level. I discontinued animal fats such as beef, steak, butter, bacon, eggs and yellow cheese and reduced the fat in my milk from 2 percent to 1 percent. On my cholesterol check at the next six-month visit to my doctor, the cholesterol level had dropped from 200 to 150 and my triglycerides to 100 which are the new normal. So, my special prior diet was not affected by my current diet which was simply using smaller and fewer portions of my customary food but remaining off the animal fats.

The only way that weight loss is sustained, is to continue the dietary selections with portion control and not return to your previous eating habits. Our method is easy to follow indefinitely since, so far, we have not limited any specific food.

Lose the weight, and THEN reconsider the other factors, based on the beneficial results of normal BMI. Be wary of any diet promotions that say never eat a particular food without verification from your physician or dietician. This type of pandering contributes to the obesity epidemic despite the thousands of diets on the market.

The specialty diets for a specific disease becomes important after completing your initial goal of a normal BMI, the starting point for a healthy mind and body, the good life with longevity.

Since I was already on a low-fat diet and was avoiding sweets and desserts, there were no further changes that I would encounter for my infirmities.

CHAPTER 8

DISEASES RELATED TO DIETS

Self-Care is increasingly important.

Understanding Your Disease even before You See Your Doctor or Dietician

As healthcare becomes more expensive, self-care is becoming more important. It is projected that Medicare and Medicaid will collapse in our lifetime. Self-care can increase in an educated society, especially with the help of the internet. One can click on almost any disease and study the medical information: causes, symptoms, diagnosis and treatment. Much of the treatment of common diseases can be undertaken initially without a prescription from or the surveillance of physicians.

A. Obesity

Obesity is one of our most common diseases. This has been explored and treatment outlined in the first six chapters of this handbook. Obesity in turn is related to other diseases which are discussed in this chapter.

Many people use medications to lose or control weight. However, they generally result in a temporary weight loss and in rebound weight gain.

There has been a current interest in weight loss surgery; but surgery seriously distorts your basic gastro-intestinal anatomy by rearranging your gastro-intestinal organs. The surgeon partially bypasses your stomach, duodenum and portions of your jejunum; nourishing food passes on to the large bowel and rectum to be evacuated from your body before all the calories and nutrients can be absorbed. Subsequent loss of vitamins and minerals may make you a slave to supplements and subject to serious nutritional disorders.

We have seen numerous patients for pre-op evaluation for surgery or banding the stomach to make it smaller. That requires an evaluation of both heart and lung risks since obesity creates difficulty in breathing. The request for evaluation of surgery risk usually states that we must have the patient lose the first 50 pounds. Why not proceed to 100 pounds? Or 200 pounds if needed to return to a normal weight. Why not arrest or cure the disease without surgery!

Self-care is also extremely important in disease prevention and the understanding of it both before and after we see our physician.

Among the Japanese, who eat little fat of any kind, breast and colon cancers are uncommon. Studies have shown that when a diet contains high amounts of fat and cholesterol, intestinal bacteria break down these foodstuffs by chemical reactions that may result in the formation of substances that act similarly to female sex hormones. Since such high fat diets usually contain little bulky, fibrous foods, the stool tends to be concentrated and to stay longer than usual in the colon; there is more exposure to carcinogens. They may stimulate the growth of cancers in hormone-sensitive tissues, such as the breast and endometrium (the lining of the uterus).

B. Diabetes Mellitus

There is a high correlation of diabetes with obesity. Today, we frequently make the diagnosis of Diabetes Mellitus before there are any sugar abnormalities in your blood. Early intervention and implementation with diet and weight control is the best and probably only way to reduce the horrendous complications that diabetes causes.

Diabetes destroys microcirculation of blood causing:

1) Retinopathy and blindness, 2) kidney failure (uremia), which then may cause hypertension and strokes, and 3) peripheral neuropathy or loss of sensation in the hands and feet, which results in injuries, cuts, bruises and infections from trauma which isn't felt; and loss of circulation which may progress to gangrene and amputations.

Therefore, many physicians consider that diabetes is the worst cardiovascular disease that humans acquire. The good news is that it can be controlled or ameliorated through early diagnosis, initiation of weight control and a low carbohydrate and sugar free diet, in association with a good exercise program started early in life. By starting this early in life, or when we first note a small amount of bulge around our middle, we can stem the tide to obesity and the numerous debilitating complications that it causes.

Blood testing kits for finger stick testing of blood sugars are OTC (over-the-counter) and quite reasonably priced at the discount houses.

There are about 18-20 million Americans who have diabetes and another 5-6 million are unaware that they have diabetes. There are also about 40-45 million Americans who have pre-diabetes, most of whom are unaware of their precarious status. Their disease is related to their genes and obesity and eating habits. These nearly 50 million can benefit the most from this handbook by checking to find if anyone has diabetes in their family. That increases their risk of developing it as well as the other members of the family. You should do them a favor by providing them a copy of this handbook which then may even prevent them from developing the disease.

The complications of diabetes can be silent and even severe before it is discovered. We have made the diagnosis of diabetes in patients with already diminished vision due to retinopathy; those with peripheral neuropathy because they've lost feeling in their fingers and toes; and those with advanced diabetic kidney disease.

This handbook will help you explore these risk factors; perhaps explode a few myths, even save your life; or avoid the suffering from all the side effects as you revise your life style.

Many times, a patient will state that one of their parents have diabetes. It is important to then explore the family history in more detail. For instance, a 30-year-old patient came in who was over-weight by 50 pounds. Both parents had diabetes and all three sisters had diabetes. She did not understand that even though her blood sugars were normal, she had preclinical or congenital diabetes mellitus.

If we have inherited a tendency to develop diabetes from our father and from our mother, we have congenital pre-diabetes even though the diabetes may be pre-clinical (before any clinical tests are positive) and remain dormant for years, and blood sugar may be normal for years.

We made the diagnosis of pre-diabetes in this patient from her family history. She, without question, had congenital pre-diabetes also. It was extremely important for her to reduce her weight to normal, eliminate simple sugars from her diet, and start an exercise program to help delay the progression to clinical diabetes.

This patient was given the list of foods for diabetics to avoid (see Appendix Two), and to obtain a glucometer, which is available OTC in any pharmacy. This is helpful in monitoring which foods may cause elevation of glucose and then avoid those foods. Patients will frequently find that after eating a large baked potato or other starchy foods for dinner, the morning fasting glucose level is rising to near 126 or higher which is the current level for the diagnosis of diabetes. Once the diagnosis of diabetes is made, most doctors will want to check their A-1c hemoglobin every six to twelve months to monitor the disease. Her more sophisticated diabetic test, the A-1c Hemoglobin was already abnormal and thus she did indeed have clinical diabetes. (The A-1c Hemoglobin has largely replaced the 4-hour glucose tolerance testing for diagnosis.) Hence, she was now at risk for all the complications of diabetes.

If, however, you don't control the intake of carbohydrates like sugar, starchy vegetables, and grains, and you frequently overload your pancreas to its maximal production of insulin, and then one day should you have a large sweet roll and sugar soaked cereal for breakfast and cake or pie alamode after dinner, it may add up to be more sugar than the secretion of insulin from your pancreas can provide to keep your glucose normal. The high carbohydrate food goes into your stomach and duodenum; the pancreas gets the message and begins working overtime churning out as much insulin as it can. But if it is not enough to keep your blood sugar normal, your blood sugar may go above 126 mg percent, the current threshold for diagnosis of diabetes. You have now confirmed that your preclinical diabetes, of which you may have been unaware, has turned into full clinical diabetes and you are eligible for all its complications.

Since you have had a high probability of diabetes since birth, this can lead to unsuspected and undiagnosed silent disease with a long latency for the complications of diabetes to form prior to when the clinical diagnosis is made.

We frequently make the diagnosis of peripheral neuropathy when a patient has numbness in the toes or fingers, a frequent complication of diabetes, and if a family history of diabetes is present, we make a tentative diagnosis of probable pre-diabetes. It is then important to implement the entire diabetic program to avoid the development of further complications. This handbook will give you directions on the required steps to delay the onset of diabetes or even possibly avoiding the full diagnosis.

In these scenarios, this handbook is critical, not only for your future health but also for your children and family in general. If there is a family history of diabetes, you may want to order several copies to give to every member of your family. It may reduce the suffering from one of mankind's most serious epidemic diseases, which has a number of significant and painful complications as outlined. It may save their lives.

Diabetes is projected to involve up to half of the population in time. At that time—some economists predict—both the Medicare and Medicaid programs will be insolvent.

There are other causes which destroy the pancreas and cause diabetes. Agent Orange in Vietnam veterans is an example of a cause of diabetes when neither parent nor any family member has had diabetes.

Destruction of the pancreas from Cancer may also destroy the Islet cells in the pancreas which produce the insulin necessary to control the blood sugar.

C. Hypertension

Essential hypertension is elevated blood pressures without apparent cause. A high sodium intake is generally believed to increase the risk of having high blood pressure. Renal hypertension is related to kidney disease which is frequently due to Diabetes and is frequently referred as DKD. (Diabetic Kidney Disease)

It is estimated that half of the adults in the United States are "at risk" of developing high blood pressure. Untreated hypertension can lead to stroke, kidney failure, heart attack and heart failure.

In 2017, the American College of Cardiology and American Heart Association acting for the first time in 14 years, redefined high blood pressure as a reading of 130 over 80, down from 140 over 90. This change means that 46 percent of U.S. adults, many of them under the age of 45, now will be considered as hypertensive, rather than "at risk" for hypertension. Robert Carey, co-chairman of the group that produced the new report. "The risk hasn't changed. What's changed is our recognition of the risk."

One of the complications of diabetes mellitus is kidney disease which in turn can be the cause of hypertension. In either case, the initial treatment is the reduction of salt in the diet. List of foods that contain significant salt are available and are noted in Appendix Five for your initial implementation even prior to seeing your doctor.

Blood pressure booths are available in most pharmacies. If your blood pressure is elevated, blood pressure measuring devices are readily available in most pharmacies. The modern wrist cuffs fit directly over the radial artery, which is the common site that doctors and nurses check your pulse and can be used to check your blood pressure. It is also small enough to fit in suitcases and overnight bags. These devices also record your BP measurements in memory, so you can take them to your physician to be recorded directly into your medical record. Some cardiologists feel that the wrist BP cuff is less accurate than the large upper arm cuff. In our experience if one places the small wrist cuff over a palpable radial artery it is as reproducible as the large cuff which frequently is not directly over the brachial artery.

* * * * *

49

Patient Anecdote/Tragedy

We saw a 44 year-old-patient who had previously experienced a stroke with aphasia (one side paralyzed with inability to speak). He had lost his insurance and ran out of his blood pressure medication. His blood pressure had gone to 240/120 according to the family before the stroke occurred. A common reason given for lack of care is "lack of insurance." This excuse is not valid. The treatment of hypertension is very cheap. Diuretics and beta-blockers cost $4 a month at the discount houses and $10 for a 3-month supply. A refillable prescription can easily be obtained from any urgent care center for a year's supply at less than the cost of an office visit. Thus, he could have avoided a life-time of total disability which included lack of communicating with his family and friends and even requiring the wheel-chair. However, his paralysis and aphasia are now permanent. He was not given any rehabilitation program by the hospital. In the short office visits I was able to teach him a word or two on each visit. This was a new experience for his brother and mother. They stated that they would continue to work on his rehabilitation.

Lack of insurance cannot be blamed for this man's severe disability with hypertension being a known easily treatable condition. With government health-care, people forget how to use private healthcare which many times is vastly cheaper. Responsible self-care is always important, whether it is done before seeing a doctor or after the patients are no longer covered by insurance.

D. Hyperlipidemia

Hyperlipidemia includes elevated triglycerides and cholesterol. Either are risk factors for cardiac and other vascular diseases. To reduce the risk for heart attacks and strokes requires a diet that avoids saturated fats. Food lists concerning those with high fat content are readily available and one is recorded in Appendix III.

In general, the animal fats are the primary ones to be avoided. When my cholesterol reached 220 mg% and my triglycerides were at 180 mg%, my doctor placed me on one of the statin drugs. In nine months my cholesterol was reduced to 200 mg% and my triglycerides to 160 mg%, but I had developed severe leg cramps, which is one of the complications of statins. This is at times caused by Rhabdomyolysis (muscle destruction) releasing myoglobin, which like hemoglobin, can cause kidney failure. A second drug caused the same side effect within one week. Rather than to try other lipid reducing drugs, I requested that my doctor give me the chance to lower my lipids with diet. This involved reducing animal fats. I eliminated beef, bacon, yellow cheese, butter, and reduced the fat in milk to 1%, and my eggs to one per week. In six months, my cholesterol was reduced to 150mg% and my triglycerides to 100mg% which some cardiologists consider the desired new normal.

My doctor honored my request for an exercise ECHO-Cardiogram which was nearly perfect. My cardiology consultant estimated my chance for a heart attack was less than 2% over the next five years. He suggested a follow up ECHO at that time. However, my personal physician stated this was not necessary. Now 20 years later, I realize this was a cost-effective decision on his part.

E. Gout

Gout is a metabolic disease with severe intermittent inflammatory joint pain and an elevated uric acid in the blood. The high levels of uric acid in the blood cause crystals to form and accumulate around a joint.

Uric acid is produced when the body breaks down a chemical called purine. Purine occurs naturally in your body, but it's also found in certain foods. Avoid meats such as liver, kidney and sweetbreads, which have high purine levels and contribute to high blood levels of uric acid. Avoid the following types of seafood, which are higher in purines than others: anchovies, herring, sardines, mussels, scallops, trout, haddock, mackerel and tuna. Beer has high purine content and is associated with an increased risk of gout and recurring attacks.

The normal level of Uric acid is < 6 mg%. With gout the levels will be at >8 mg% or greater.

A low-purine gout diet may help decrease uric acid levels in the blood. While not a cure, it may lower the risk of recurring painful gout attacks and slow the progression of joint damage. Medication also is used to manage pain and to lower levels of uric acid.

Gout is readily treated with Colchicine for the gout attacks and Allopurinol to reduce the level of uric acid. By avoiding food high in purines, the uric acid can be reduced to normal. However, it may be wise to keep some colchicine on hand in your medicine cabinets in case you have a gout attack which can be very severe and painful.

F. Osteoporosis

Osteoporosis, the loss of bone density is increasingly common with age. Risk factors include genetics, lack of exercise, lack of calcium and vitamin D, personal history of fracture as an adult, cigarette smoking, excessive alcohol consumption, history of rheumatoid arthritis, low body weight, and family history of osteoporosis. Patients with osteoporosis have no symptoms until bone fractures occur. The diagnosis of osteoporosis can be suggested by X-rays and confirmed by tests to measure bone density.

Bone is living, growing tissue. Throughout life our bodies are breaking down old bone and rebuilding new bone in a continuous cycle. Bones progressively increase in density until a maximum level is reached, usually around age 30.

We gain bone by building more than we lose. After about age 35, this balance begins to reverse with bone loss beginning to occur at a slightly faster rate than it can be replaced, which causes bones to slowly decrease in density and to become more brittle.

Bones contain minerals such as calcium and phosphorus, which make them hard and dense. To maintain bone density, the body requires an adequate supply of calcium, and vitamin D3 along with proper amounts of several hormones, such as parathyroid hormone, growth hormone, calcitonin, estrogen in women, and testosterone in men. Healthy bone also requires adequate physical exercise. That is why osteoporosis is seen in weightlessness as in astronauts.

After menopause and the loss of estrogen, bones' inner mesh becomes increasingly thinner, weaker and more brittle. But it is only when bone loss is excessive, as can be measured by a bone density scan, for example, that a person would be diagnosed with osteoporosis.

The most common problem associated with osteoporosis is bone fractures; the bones of the wrist, spine and hip are the most likely to break. Hip fractures are the most serious as they can lead to long-term hospitalization, permanent disability and loss of independence. Unfortunately, after one osteoporotic fracture, others are more likely to follow. Besides that, fractures tend to heal slowly in those who suffer with osteoporosis.

Don't wait for your doctor to prescribe a walker to help you prevent falls, fractures, and a lifetime of disability. You should get your walker immediately after your first fall. You can order it from the internet at one-fourth of what Medicare would pay. Or you could order it from your nearest medical supply house. You shouldn't wait until you get Medicare approval, which could be too late. If you wait until after your second fall and get a fracture you could end up with long-term disability and perhaps never walk again.

G. Heart Disease

Heart attacks are the leading cause of death and illness in the United States. In coronary atherosclerosis and coronary thrombosis, there is the accumulation of "plaque" (cholesterol, fatty deposits, and other substances) on the inner lining of coronary walls. This buildup narrows the coronary arteries until they become so clogged that blood cannot flow through. This may result in coronary ischemia with damage to part of the heart muscle that it supplies.

Many factors are associated with heart disease. For example, a smoker has a statistically greater chance of developing cardiovascular disease and dying of a heart attack or stroke than does a nonsmoker. Other factors associated with greater risk are obesity, hypertension, high cholesterol, and diabetes.

Therefore, this entire handbook is important in reducing heart disease. Read and digest it well.

PART II –PHYSICAL EXERCISE

CHAPTER 9

HEALTH ASSESSMENT OVERVIEW

Your Exercise Program

We have gone over the rules of eating for achieving your ideal weight. We trust you are well on your way to a normal BMI. But this may not fully provide optimal mental, physical health or well-being. One can have a normal BMI with the muscles, joints and ligaments in an uncoordinated or weakened state. This then leads to a number of serious disabilities. Just missing a step from the curb, you can dislocate, injure or tear a ligament or muscle that is not in an optimal condition. For a healthy mind and body, you will need a total body reconditioning program.

Although it's difficult to pinpoint one factor that has the greatest effect on health and longevity, according to the U.S. Centers for Disease Control (CDC), physical activity is one of the most important factors in maintaining health. People who are physically active tend to live longer and have a lower risk of many chronic health conditions, such as heart disease, Type 2 diabetes, depression, traumatic injuries such as sprains, dislocations, fractures, and some cancers. Evidence is also beginning to show physical activity is associated with a delay in onset of deteriorating mental and neurologic conditions.

Total body reconditioning will include a normal BMI, or an active progression to a normal BMI; maintaining ROM by daily morning stretch/flex to tune up your muscles, tendons, and joint ligaments that you will be using all day; and then aerobic exercises with the accepted standard of 150 minutes per week. Jogging, running or even fast walking is acceptable. And then a muscle development program to increase strength to facilitate physical work throughout the day.

Physical activity is beneficial to people of all ages and fitness levels, stresses the CDC. Further, a combination of aerobic exercise, muscle-strengthening exercise and bone-and joint-strengthening exercise is scientifically proven to slow the loss of bone density that comes with advancing age. Exercise helps alleviate the pain of arthritis for many people and decreases the risk of hip fracture in older adults. For example, moderate-intensity aerobic activity such as jogging 75 minutes per week also helps many adults maintain a healthy weight. If the above exercise is not attainable because of age other infirmity, people who are moderately active for at least 7 hours per week (One hour per day) are 40 percent less likely to die early than those who are active for 30 minutes per week or less—but 5 minutes a day doesn't do it.

Physical activity also offers mental health benefits. The Mental Health Foundation points out that when you exercise it causes the brain to release chemicals known as endorphins responsible for improving mood. Even a brisk, 10-minute walk improves alertness, energy and feelings of well-being.

Furthermore, a combination of 30 to 60 minutes of aerobic and muscle-strengthening activities three to five times per week helps maintain balance, strength, thinking, judgement and learning skills as people age, according to the CDC.

Executives working at a desk doing significant strenuous mental activity, who frequently recognize mental fatigue by mid-afternoon, state that going out for a 10- or 15-minute brisk walk renews their mental capacities and they accomplish more. A Silicon Valley entrepreneur stated that when he notes he's not accomplishing much by midafternoon he drives out to his private plane and roams around the sky for 30 minutes and is amazingly refreshed when he delves into his work again.

Muscle and joint strengthening exercises are also important. This would include the ROM of each joint daily. The pushups, sit-ups, barbell lifting, and deep knee bending can all be done at home.

Your Personal Exercise Program:

If you've joined an exercise gym, it is easy to transfer your entire fitness program to your home. All you need is a bench press available from any sports store and a foam pad next to it for your pushups and sit-ups. These are readily available for less cost than three-month dues in a gym. They only require a space approximated 8 x 8 foot in the garage or spare bedroom. Taking a walk outdoors is as effective as a treadmill and considerably more refreshing and healthy. With your fast walk, be sure to take a small felt covered barbell in each hand and raise your forearm at least 45-90 degrees with each step so you condition your wrist, forearms, upper arms and shoulders as you walk. Also raise your shoulders slightly to help condition your shoulder girdle. The legs and thighs get the same treatment just from the fast walk. Women will normally start with a one-pound barbell in each hand and men with a two-pound barbell in each hand. You can progress along your series of barbells as desired or able.

We will look at the three components of a health exercise program in the next three chapters:

A. The Morning Stretch/Flex

The Morning Stretch/Flex routine helps develop the full ROM and function of every joint in your body. This tunes up your muscles, tendons and the ligaments in your joints and only takes about 5 minutes. It can best be done the first thing in the morning in your bedroom, preferably in front of a mirror which helps you achieve the maximal stretch. Since we use our muscles and joints daily in any activity, this should be done seven days a week. It can also easily be done while at a business meeting or on a vacation. It can also be repeated during the day when prolonged inactivity causes muscle and joint aches and pains.

B. The Aerobics

Aerobics, which includes running, jogging or fast walking, are the most important factor in maintaining mental and physical abilities throughout life. They can be done in the mornings after your Stretch/Flex routine or any time during the day while on a work break or in the evening after work in your neighborhood and takes approximately 25 minutes a day, six days a week. Rest on your Holy day. Use the same barbell for your aerobics that you used for the Stretch/Flex routine to help condition your upper extremities while the running, jogging or fast walking conditions your lower body.

C. Muscle, Tendon & Ligament Strengthening

The strengthening exercise is sometimes called your workout and makes all your physical work more efficient. It also helps prevent injuries and fractures. This is best done with a bench press to develop your upper and lower extremities at the same time. Use a foam pad for your pushups and sit-ups. In the absence of a bench press, barbell weights can be used.

CHAPTER 10

THE MORNING STRETCH/FLEX

Daily Routine

Tune up your muscle, tendons, joints and ligaments daily.

Before you exercise or progress to physical work, it is important to prepare your joints and muscles through a ROM (range of motion) routine also called the morning Stretch/Flex, to warm up all the muscle groups, joints, tendons, and ligaments for optimal function. This is very important for avoiding strains and sprains or even a fracture. All joints have muscles that move the joint. A hinge type of joint, such as your elbow and knee, will move in two directions. While one set of muscles flex to move the joint, the other set is stretched in the same maneuver. Hence, the stretch/flex name. A ball and socket joint such as your shoulder or hip moves in all directions. So, in addition to the flex/stretch muscles, there are additional muscles to rotate your shoulder or hip. These joints need to be rotated to condition (stretch/flex) all the rotator type of muscles. Your muscles and joints should be prepared for a sudden shift in use during the day. A misstep from an uneven sidewalk or curb, if that is the first challenge of the day, may cause a severe strain or sprain of any weight bearing joint including your back. So, make sure that every muscle, tendon, joint and ligament is prepared for the day's activities as well as any unknown sudden strain even if your work is primarily considered sedentary office work. Inappropriate lifting or carrying of a printer or computer when your job classification may be sedentary or light work could cause a sudden strain or pinched nerve not normally considered a risk in this sort of job.

On every physical examination that I've done during my 45 years of medical practice, not only did I examine the head, eyes, ears, nose, throat, heart, lungs, and abdomen, I also did an orthopedic and a neurologic exam. Patients were impressed. On their way out of the office they would tell my wife at the front desk that they had never had such a thorough examination. It was the orthopedic/neurological portion of the exam, I believe, that primarily impressed them. It is one portion of the annual exam in which the patient needs to actively participate. I recommend doing this range of motion (ROM) at home every morning, preferably three times for each joint. I find it important to walk a patient through this routine, simply explaining does not yield results.

The Range of Motion (ROM) Exam

This is the first part of the orthopedic portion of a general physical examination and is basically a mobility exam of all the joints in the body. If the ROM is normal for a joint, it is more likely than not that the joint will be normal. The patient must be standing and facing the examiner. A physician's medical ortho exam would entail the measured or estimation of the ROM of each joint. The physician would normally do this once for each joint and record the result. If abnormal, the physician may have you repeat it once or twice to make sure he's recording the maximum ROM.

For your own stretch/flex exam, it may be best to be in front of at least a half-length mirror which allows you to observe the movement of all your joints and muscles. This is a warm up of the entire musculo-skeletal system of your body. Each joint should be examined to the maximum ROM three times every morning. Once is just the initial stretch/flex but doing each a second or third time will improve the range to the maximum. The normal ROMs are recorded below. If you can't reach the normal, this indicates that you needed the three tries to push each joint to the maximum. (Professional athletes and body builders will do these 50 to 100 times once or twice a day.)

The Spine Stretch/Flex ROM

We normally begin with the axial skeleton which is the cervical, thoracic, lumbar and sacral spine. The spine is a series of bones, muscles, ligaments, tendons which houses the spinal cord which receives information from the brain and sends messages to the entire body through a system of peripheral nerves. It also gives messages back to the brain in reflex fashion or as information to allow your brain to respond after receiving the message. The spine is a series of bones called vertebrae which are hooked together by facets with a cartilaginous disk between them. The nerves exit the spinal cord protected by this disc. When this disc is damaged through heavy lifting or trauma, the bony spine may pinch the nerves causing severe pain to the portion of the body that it serves. The bony spine or vertebrae are encased by large para spinal muscles that support the spine. Without the large supporting muscles, the spine would not remain upright. Keeping these large muscles in good condition is extremely important in preventing backaches and pains radiating into the arms and legs.

The spine moves in all directions. Therefore, to determine its ROM function, we must move it in four directions plus rotate both ways: flexing/stretching in all four directions and rotation in two. This includes forward bending, backward bending, and sideways bending to the left and to the right and rotation to the left and to the right. These can be done in any order.

The Cervical Spine ROM. (The Stretch/Flex of the Neck)

We begin at the first portion of the spine which is the cervical portion or the neck. To check the ROM in all directions, we put our chin on our chest or sternum, and then arch our necks backwards as far as possible. Do these three times to achieve the maximal ROM. This forward and backward stretch/flexion should be 45-degrees. We then put our left ear to our left shoulder and our right ear to our right shoulder. This is lateral flexion and should also be 45-degrees. This should be repeated for three stretches to achieve our maximum stretch and flexion. We then rotate our neck by putting our chin to each shoulder which should be about 80 degrees. If you can only do 60 or 75 degrees, try to push it slightly each day to see if you can reach normal. Repeat these three times. Some of the muscles are attached to the shoulder and the ROM should be checked again three times with your shoulders elevated to increase flexibility and engage shoulder muscles.

This will be very important in keeping our necks mobile and fully functional. The neck is a very common cause of disability and doing this daily may prevent disability and a life of pain. A pinched nerve in the neck may send a sharp electrical pain into the arms which will represent the distribution of that cervical nerve. This is called radiculopathy. As that nerve is damaged and causes loss of sensation or function, it is called neuropathy or neuropathic pain. Your physician maps this out in the neurologic exam which accompanies every orthopedic and neurologic exam.

The Thoracic-Lumbar-Sacral Spine

The stretch/flex of the back also called the Dorsal Spine and sometimes is called the lumbo-sacral spine. The ROM stretch/flexion here is essentially the same that was done to the C-Spine. These can be done in any order.

To begin with rotation, rotate your shoulders three times, this rotates your spine to 90-degrees in each direction. Normal is 80 degrees but most of us can do 90 degrees. Then bend to the right and to the left three times. This should be 30 degrees or more of lateral flexion. Then bend backwards to 30 degrees and then forward to 90 degrees three times. If you cannot reach your toes, just bend several times until you come close to your toes. This will determine if your vertebral joints are in good health and will stretch your muscles and associated ligaments. Doing each of these three times can help to prevent backaches and sprains. Your physician will normally do this once and estimate your ROM for your medical record.

People with chronic back problems say that the spinal ROM has been the most helpful in preventing or in alleviating their back pain. If you start this at an early age, you may never develop backache pains unless you have an injury. Doing this ROM is an easy way to prevent disability and a life of pain.

A pinched nerve here is essentially the same process as the pinched nerve in the cervical spine and may cause lumbar radiculopathy down the path of that nerve. When there is destruction of that nerve, it progresses to lumbo-sacral neuropathy or neuropathic pain. Your physician will map this area in the neurologic exam which accompanies every orthopedic exam.

During my ortho exam on patients, I would do each ROM once and record the maximum. For back conditioning as part of the exercise program, one would do each ROM three times. (Professional athletes and body builders will do these 50 to 100 times once or twice a day.)

Upper Extremities (Shoulders, arms, elbows, wrist, hand and fingers)

Our Shoulders are ball and socket joints and thus must function in all directions. We must move them also in the same six maneuvers: four flexion/extensions and two rotations. We begin by elevating our arms forward to 180 degrees and then backward to minus 45 degrees three times. We then extend our arms outwards up to 180 degrees, (which uses different muscles) and then cross them in front to 45 degrees three times. To rotate our shoulders, rotate the outstretched hand from palm up to palm down positions three times and repeat with elbows bent at 90 degrees outward. To tone up your rotator cuff tendons, move the hands to the middle of your spine near the shoulders blades and rotate again from your hands three times. Women seldom have rotator cuff tears since they do this every time they get dressed. Men have them more frequently since they don't exercise their rotator cuffs when getting dressed. Most men now-a-days have tossed the wash cloth and use a hand towel to be able to wash their backs.

Personal Experience

I tore my rotator cuff when suddenly reaching from the front seat to the back seat of my car to acquire an object. It was obvious that I'd torn my left rotator cuff ligament. I never saw an orthopedist for a confirmatory diagnosis and therefore did not obtain an MRI. I was unable to remove my billfold from my left back pocket for about six months while waiting for it to heal. Rotator cuff injuries obviously have occurred for

63

thousands of years and nature healed most of them. It just became a surgical opportunity in the 20th century. Thus, I saved Medicare at least $10,000 to $15,000. Avoidance of unnecessary surgery is another way to reduce our nation's health care costs.

* * * * *

Surgical Anecdote

I saw one patient who had a shoulder rotator cuff tear and went to an orthopedic surgeon because that was the customary thing. He did an arthroscopic exam and repair through a small incision into her joint. Afterwards her pain was worse. The orthopedist stated that he would have to go in again and clean it out more thoroughly. She followed his recommendations. When she came back, she stated that the pain was even worse. We tried to manage the pain for her. After two more years of suffering, she finally said, the pain was so severe that she went back to the same orthopedist a third time, signing another permit for a third arthroscopic surgical procedure. This time he placed metal hardware in her joint including screws to secure her tendons to the bone. When she came back again, she complained of having even more pain. How much? She estimated the pain was at least a hundred times worse than before the first operation. Surgery isn't always the best option, except, perhaps for the surgeon.

We frequently are asked to clear a patient for surgery. Surgeons want to know if their patient will survive the operation. Therefore, we have had the opportunity to observe these patient conditions before and after surgery on hips, knees, spine and other joints as well.

* * * * *

Comparing the medical and surgical specialties with the occupational skilled trades

The Menninger Clinic did a study on the occupational skills trade in order to ascertain as to what other careers workers might have chosen had they proceeded to college and/or professional school. They found that Carpenters would choose orthopedic surgery should they have gone on to college and medical school. Perhaps that partially explains why orthopedists like joint reconstruction with hardware, bolts, wire, and screws.

Surgery for pain is seldom effective.

* * * * *

The **Elbows** are a hinge type of joint and thus move in only two directions: Extension and flexion. The **Ulna** bone in our forearm is the hinged joints and only move in two directions. We extend our forearms out to 180 degrees (straight) and flex them back to 145 degrees three times. The **Radius** is the other bone in the forearm, which goes from the wrist to the elbow where it rotates. It is controlled by the hand and examined by palm up and palm down maneuvers which rotates the radius. This should also be done three times.

To check our **Wrists**, we bend our hands downward 80 degrees and upward 70 degrees. We flex our wrists to the thumb side by 20 degrees and to the small finger side by 45 degrees. Do each three times.

We then extend and flex our **Fingers** and **Thumb** maximally by spreading our fingers as well as making a fist. The extension should be 180 degrees or straight. On flexion, the first joint should be 90 degrees and the second joint 100 degrees. On full flexion as in making a fist, the tips of our fingers should go to the transverse crease in our palms. If they don't, just use the other hand to force them a bit closer. Doing these three times each day maintains the finger joints ROM and finger flexibility.

Lower Extremities (Hips, Thighs, Knees, Ankles, Feet and Toes.)

Hips are another **Ball and Socket** joint. So, we flex them in all four directions and then rotate them in both directions for the same six maneuvers. We bring our knees to our chest to flex the hips 130 degrees. We then bring our legs 30 degrees backward which extends the hips. We then move our legs outward 45 degrees which is a motion in our hips and then bring them inward across the midline to 20 degrees. We rotate our hips by toeing out 60 degrees and toeing in 30 degrees. Do all three ROM three times for each hip.

We can repeat this during the course of our day to improve ROM that is limited. For instance, we can do this by crossing our legs. A good stretch for rotating our hips is to place the foot or ankle on the opposite knee while sitting and then pushing the knee downward with our hand. This will stretch the ligaments in the hip joint and further condition them. This is an exercise we can do frequently during the day whether we're sitting in our homes, at work, or in an auditorium. This helps prevent ankylosis or a frozen hip which may also cause difficulty or even prevent a female from engaging in sexual intercourse.

Knees are a hinge join and hence move only in two directions. To check the ROM, we straighten our legs to 180 degrees extension or fully straightened. Then we flex our legs backwards to 140 degrees. Do these three times. Since this is a hinge joint, any movement sideways reflects damaged knee ligaments.

Knee ligaments can best be strengthened by deep knee bends, walking or running. Also, a small bench press at home has a knee function setting similar to what orthopedists use when strengthening the knee ligaments post-surgery. On your personal bench press, you can strengthen your knee ligaments at the same time you are doing your arm and shoulder strengthening maneuvers.

To check our **Ankles**, we raise our heel by standing on our toes and the foot should be at an angle of 45 degrees. (Women can measure how far this places the heel above floor level. If this is approximate four or five inches, then women should be comfortable in a three-inch heel without any undue strain on their ankle.) We then stand on our heels raising our forefoot up which should be at an angle of 20 degrees. Then invert the foot inward for 30 degrees and evert our foot outward by 20 degrees. Do these ROM three times. This helps to prevent a sprained ankle.

Checking the **Toes** requires bare feet. Thus, it is best to do this in the morning Stretch/Flex routine before you get dressed and put on your shoes. If you missed, do this in the evening when you remove them. Bend your toes upwards maximally and feel free to help with your hands with a slight stretch. Toes can also be stretched by kneeling with the toes bent forward. Bending them down requires placing the foot on a ledge and try for 90-degree flexion. A large book or dictionary may help. Or one can proceed while kneeling and bending the toes backwards. Occasionally the last joint of a toe, frequently the second and/or the third toe, will bend downward and not fully straighten. This is called a hammer toe. If it's totally frozen (ankylosed) a podiatrist may have to cut the tendons to allow full extension. However, if you note this is starting to happen, just manually stretch that last joint and straighten it and hold if for a few minutes each day. This can easily be done before putting on your shoes or anytime you're sitting with bare feet. This will completely prevent a hammer toe ankylosis and the difficulty in wearing shoes.

CONGRATULATIONS!

You have now checked all your joints and hopefully, they should have a normal range of motion or be on a track for full ROM. Do these stretch/flex exercises for each joint three times every morning to keep all your joint, tendons and muscles stretched and the internal ligaments active, and thereby, keep your joints in good health and help prevent injuries. Do this daily, seven days a week to keep all your joints mobile for life. This should take about five minutes every morning in front of a mirror before getting dressed to help gage how complete your ROMs are. This can be repeated at any time during the day whenever you feel stiff or achy and usually results in immediate improvement. (Athletes and body builders do all the above 50 to 100 times once or twice daily, so they can use their muscle, tendon, joints, and ligaments maximally.)

Caveat:

Doing the ROM with a one- or two-pound barbell in each hand will help you proceed to full body reconditioning more rapidly. Women will usually begin with a one-pound barbell in each hand and men will normally start with a two-pound barbell in each hand. Extra maneuvers during your work day, such as deep knee bends, standing on your toes, your heels, crossing your legs and pushing the knee downward while ankle on opposite knee will keep your hips, knees, ankles and feet moving smoothly for years longer.

CHAPTER 11

HEALTH BENEFITS OF EXERCISE

Exercise and Aerobic Physical Activity

Exercise contributes to both physical and mental well-being. Regular physical activity is one of the most important things you can do for your health. Aerobic exercises are a most important factor in maintaining mental and physical abilities throughout life.

Fitness means being able to perform physical activity. It also means having the energy and strength to feel as good as possible and improve your health. Your heart, your brain, muscles, joints, and metabolism, essentially your entire body, benefit from exercise.

Enrollment in the physical fitness programs is very popular. Gyms are sprouting up all over. There are four within walking distance of my home. However, few of my neighbors walk to their gyms. They drive their cars just to go a few blocks. The data indicates that only about 82 percent of those fitness gym members make use of it daily. There are 17 new gyms in Sacramento, which are part of a national chain. They bemoan that only 8 percent of their members achieve their initial goals. It seems to have been reduced to an expensive status symbol. Yet use has decreased because it becomes a hassle to go over to the gym daily. It also takes much longer to go to and from the gym than it would if you exercised at home. Doing these exercises at home and in your neighborhood helps to make exercise a significant part of your daily life for the rest of your life.

Exercise increases muscle mass, which is 50 percent heavier than the fat mass it replaces. However it has to be primarily aerobic exercise to be effective. The accepted amount of baseline aerobics is 150 minutes per week. This can be done three days a week for 50 minutes each day or it can be in six days for 25 minutes a day. Running or jogging is considered the basic aerobic exercises.

A fast walk qualifies as aerobic, especially if you have a small barbell in each hand moving in sync with your legs. This engages the muscles of the arms, hands, elbows and shoulders. Walking engages the muscles and joints of the feet, legs, thighs and pelvis.

Women are generally comfortable starting with a one-pound weight in each hand progressing to a two-pound weight in three to six months. We've observed some women will progress to a three-pound barbell in each hand during their fast walk at the one-year point.

Men should start with a two-pound barbell in each hand and generally progress to a three-pound weight in three to six months. They may progress to four-pounds in six months. Some men progress to a five-pound barbell within one year.

Be sure to partially raise your arms to 60-90 degrees during each fast walk and move them from side-to-side to activate the muscles in your wrist, forearm, arm and shoulder as you walk. Also raise your shoulders for portions of your aerobic activity to further condition your shoulder muscles. This will condition your upper extremities while the walking conditions your lower extremities. The twisting motion from side-to-side will also help to keep your back muscles in good condition.

Barbells come in single handed neoprene or felt-covered models to be used in each hand while doing the fast walk or jogging. Thus, the investment in a pair of a one-, two-, three-four- and five-pound set of barbells will normally be adequate for an entire family for both the Stretch/Flex as well as the Aerobic portion of this reconditioning program.

The usual walk is 3 mph or a mile in 20 minutes. The fast walk must be at least 4 mph or a mile in 15 minutes. If you use a pedometer, an iPhone, or an iPod for measurements, you may have to readjust the distance since these instruments measure steps. Since we know there are 880-yards in a half mile and 1760 yards for a mile, by measuring your steps you can make a quick calculation of how many steps equal a half or a full mile. My iPod registers 2200 steps when I walk and calls it one mile. Since my steps were approximately 30 inches, it was indeed

1760 yards or one mile. Therefore my iPod is set at about 30-inches per step or accurate enough for my program. Also try to increase the length of each step, in addition to the speed. Men can usually increase their steps to 36 inches, which I have now done, and women to 30 inches. Don't worry about converting the distance and confusing yourself. Just keep walking fast.

None of this requires the expense of belonging to an exercise club or gym or buying a treadmill. It doesn't even require getting into gym clothes. It can be done in the middle of the day at work or from a business office during lunch, or from your home in the mornings or after work.

More info: https://www.cdc.gov/physicalactivity/basics/pa-health/index.htm#LiveLonger

CHAPTER 12

MUSCLE STENGTHENING EXERCISE

Muscle, Tendon & Ligament Strengthen

You have done the first step in this exercise with the stretch/flex routine every morning as well as the second step that is your aerobic program, which helps you to be satisfied with eating less. Now we will proceed with the third part of your exercise program, the strengthening exercises.

Muscle building is not part of the weight loss program since muscles weigh more than fat, but it improves your outlook and indirectly helps your weight loss program. It is also important if your muscles are weak or markedly deconditioned to prevent falls and other injuries.

This can best be done with a bench press apparatus readily available from any sports store. There are progressive weights to strengthen your shoulders and arms as well as weights for your legs, which allow you to build them up at the same time.

It can also be done with a series of weights in barbell fashion. For decades, rows of cardio and weight machines have filled U.S. gyms like platoons of a robot army. But their ranks are thinning according to Rachel Backman in the December 2017 Wall Street Journal. Traditional health clubs are removing some machines to open floor space for small-group training.

The Bench Press

Bench presses have become affordable and are vastly cheaper than the exercise clubs. It is also nearby in your home or garage which improves usage. In our area a bench press cost is about equal to the cost of three months in the exercise parlors. Bench presses allow for muscle, joint, tendon and ligament conditioning equal to a half dozen or more machines in the exercise gyms and is equally as effective. The statistics reveal that the average regular usage of exercise gyms is about 82 percent of member enrollees. This reflects that enrollment is as much a status symbol as being interested in a healthy body and mind. If you have experience with exercise gyms and didn't make it to the gym on a regular basis, you should invest in a small bench press with a set of weights.

A small bench press has settings for lifting weights with your arms while simultaneously exercising your knees with progressive weights. This strengthens your tendons and ligaments and helps prevent tearing. This lifting of weights while on your back strengthens tendons and ligaments in the hands, forearms, upper arms and shoulders. The simultaneous lift of your legs strengthens the muscles, tendons, and ligaments in the ankles, legs, knees, thighs and hips.

Women are now competing with men in weight lifting. One of my patients, a nurse, was maximizing her lifting to become the women's weight-lifting world champion. She was up to 300-pound weights when she ruptured her biceps muscle. She never got to 300 pounds again nor became the women's world champion. Don't overdo it!

Bench Press/Gym Foam Pad

I have my bench press in the garage. When my Catera car died about 4 years ago, I decided that since my wife had a full-size Buick, I no longer needed a back seat or a trunk. I just needed half-a-car as a commuter-car from my home to my office, to the Veteran's Administration Clinic, to U.C. Davis, and to my primary hospital. All are within ten miles from my home. With a 10-foot car rather than an 18-foot car, this gave me an 8 x 8-foot area for my exercise gym. I purchased a bench press at the sports store and a foam pad. Each one takes up an adjacent area of 8 x 4 feet. My Bench Press cost me about the same as three months' dues of $85 per month at the nearby exercise facility. Some of the exercise gyms are now reducing their charges because of the competition. Meanwhile, a new system catering to women is charging $139 a month. The initial reviews indicate only an 8 percent success rate.

Push-ups and simultaneous Leg-ups

With a series of weights from 2-½, 5-, or 10-pounds on each end of the rod and 5-, 10-, or 15-pounds on the foot lift, I was essentially able to do a complete body strengthening program including knee strengthening with the weights on the foot apparatus. Start with the 2-½ pound weight on either end of the bar and lift it five times while simultaneously extending your knees with the 5-pound weight on the leg apparatus. Increase lifts every three months until you reach your goal of 100 lifts for the strengthening portion of this program. This is because it has a different progressive endpoint (muscle strengthening) than the three-time stretch/flex program (joint mobility). After you've reached your 100 lifts, increase the weight by 2-½ pounds progressing to 5-, or 10- pounds on each end of the rod if possible.

I stayed at 7-½ pounds on each end of the rod and 15 pounds on the leg lift and gradually increased the number of lifts to 200 times each day. I then increased weight on each end of the bar by 2-½ pounds (equally a total of 10 pounds) and am gradually building up to 200 pushes.

To strengthen your back, do pushups on your foam pad. Start on your knees with your fingers spread and lift your body five times which strengthens your fingers, arms, shoulders, back and legs. Increase by five push-ups every three months as you are able.

After six months, try to do the pushups from your toes. Start with five and increase by five every three months as you are able. Continue with strengthening your fingers by spreading them as you do the lifting. Whether you do pushups from your knees or from your toes, this strengthens your back muscles as well as all the muscles in your arms, shoulders, elbow, wrist and fingers. When you do the full push-ups from your toes, you also strengthen the muscles of your hips, legs, ankles, and feet. Thus, the pushups help to prevent back aches, especially from heavy lifting or prolonged sitting which is more common in the work place now. The complaints of back pain in an office work setting don't seem to be diminishing. In fact, prolong sitting causes some of the most severe back pains. Just look at the numerous ergonomic chairs that have been developed to help alleviate this. My back pains as well as the radiation of pain to my toes, have resolved with these additional push-up/sit-up exercise maneuvers.

Sit-ups

Proceed by rolling over on your back on the foam pad and do five sit-ups. Do this by lying flat on the foam pad; stretch your legs straight and your arms straight above your head. Very slowly, lift your shoulders up to a sitting position, as your arms move forward and down towards your toes. Then proceed by touching your left toes with your right fingers; and then your right toes with your left hand. Then very slowly, as you count to five, lower yourself back down on the pad into a flat position. This brings your abdominal muscles into the routine. Do these five times and increase the number by five every three to six months as possible.

Barbells

Begin with your 1-, 2-, 3-, 4-, or 5-pound barbell weight in each hand or the equivalent on a rod. Raise them from the floor to overhead height forward, hold for five seconds, and then return them slowly to the floor. Do these five times. Repeat moving weights outward from floor to 180 degrees up five times, hold five seconds, and then return them slowly to the floor. Then raise your weights 90 degrees and rotate your wrists, this rotates your shoulders. Do this five times increase the number by five every three months or as possible. Also progress to the next weight every six months as tolerated.

For muscle strengthening without a bench press, you will need to progress to the next series of barbells which are 8-, 10-, 12-, 15-, and 20-pound barbells or the equivalent on a rod. They can be neoprene or felt covered. Continue as above with this series by lifting the weights forward 180 degrees, hold for 5 seconds and then return them slowly to the floor. Then continue outward 180 degrees, hold, and then return them to the floor as before. Then raise them 90 degrees and rotate the hands. This rotates your shoulders, ball and socket joints. Do each five times and progress as possible.

Leg-ups without the bench press

The push-ups/ sit-ups are essentially the same as previously discussed. However, without the foot apparatus of the bench press, we need to add the leg-up exercise. Lying on your back on your foam pad, lift both legs 6 inches off the pad, spread them to 45 degrees, count to five, and back to the center, count to five and lower slowly to the pad. Repeat five times. The foam pad will protect any bony prominences, such as your tail bone, on a board, hardwood floor, or cement garage floor.

Deep knee bends

Stand up and do deep knee bends five times to strengthen your legs, knees, hips and thigh muscles. Squat down maximally to sit on your ankles as you progress to a standing position. Increase the number by five every three months or as possible.

You may have friends who tell you that they have an "anterior collateral ligament" tear in their knees. This is one of the first stages towards knee arthritis or degenerative joint disease (DJD). After several arthroscopies, they may notice the knees are loose and have a little sideways motion. The orthopedist will more likely than not talk them into a knee arthroplasty (Knee joint replacement) surgery. This is becoming more common. However, those of us on the medical side of the health care team that clear their patients for surgical risk, see all the failures and poor alignments. I have one patient whose toes point outwards when he walks.

Discuss possible complications with your surgeon before you sign the operative permit.

I have another patient who's had three knee replacements and now the bone cement in the tibia of the third artificial knee has come loose and the foot dangles. She's asking her orthopedic surgeon to amputate above the knee, so she can get a good solid prosthesis and walk better with less pain. Following the outline in this handbook would do much to prevent such DJD.

* * * * *

Total Body Reconditioning Program done at Home

I. Daily stretch/flex of all your joints every morning.

(5 minutes daily 7 days a week)

This is best done in AM daily, seven days a week since we use our muscles and joints daily, (even on the Holy Days,) to avoid sudden surges which may result in sprains/strains whenever we walk or miss a step. Having a one- or two-pound weight in each hand can further speed up your reconditioning. This can be repeated after prolonged 4-5 hours of sitting or sooner if you experience a backache while at work. Doing each joint three times obtains the maximal stretch/flex. We are strengthening, not muscle building, with the stretch/flex morning routine.

* * * * *

II. Aerobics: 150 minutes per week

This can be done in 25 minutes a day for 6 days a week or 50 minutes a day for three days a week. It can be as simple as jogging or a fast walk for the same period of time. Be sure to have a small one- or two-pound barbell in each hand raising it 45-90 degrees with each step to condition your upper body as you condition your lower body.

We find the six-day week routine reduces lapses.

* * * * *

III. Muscle Strengthening program

This is best done with a bench press with adjacent foam pad to strengthen the upper and lower body.

This can be done in 5-10 minutes daily six days a week.

No exercise gym or gym clothes are required.

* * * * *

With Small Bench Press

Easily acquired from your local sports store.

Upper body

Women will start with 2.5-pound weights on each end of barbell bar on the Bench Press. Increase 2.5-pound weights in six months as tolerated. No need to go further than 5-pounds if muscles fatigue occurs. For muscle strengthening we need to do five lifts and increase by five every three – six months. No upper body limits.

Men will start with a 5-pound weight on each end of the barbell bar and add 2.5-pound weights in six months if tolerated. If muscle fatigue occurs, no need to go beyond 7.5 pounds. For muscle strengthening, we need to do five lifts daily and increase by five lifts every 3-6 months. No upper limits. (Note: I maxed out at 10. When I'm up to 200 lifts per day I will progress to 12.5 pounds after that.)

Lower body

Start with 5-pound weight on the leg apparatus and increase 2.5 pounds every six months as tolerated. Repeat five times simultaneously with the arm push-ups. (I maxed out at 15 pounds when my knee ligaments became painful. They have recovered, and I may try 20 pounds again.) These are muscle strengthening exercises. Hence, no upper limits except those which are determined by you.

* * * * *

With Barbell Weights--No Bench Press

Easily acquired from your local sports store

Begin to acquire additional 8-, 10-, 15-, and 20-pound felt, or neoprene covered barbells for weight lifting and muscle strengthening exercises six days a week.

To develop your upper body

Warm up with the pair of 5-pound barbell weights, by lifting them up from the floor and over your head to 180 degrees. Hold, count to ten and lower slowly back down to the floor. Then lift them up from the floor and out to your sides to 180 degrees. Hold, count to ten and back slowly to the floor. Do each five times. Increase by five lifts every 3-6 months.

Progress to the heavier barbell series: 8-, 10-, 15-, and 20-pounds lifting and repeating both the upward and outward motions to 180 degrees. Do each five times. Increase lifts by five every 3-6 months as tolerated, or muscles become fatigued. These are your workout muscle strengthening exercises and there are no upper limits except yours. If your muscles fatigue with the 8- or 10-pound weight, don't progress but remain at that weight until you are comfortable with that weight for 25 to 50 lifts and then proceed to the next in the series.

To develop your lower body

Begin by lying on your back, raise your legs straight out and up six inches, hold (count to 10), spread to 45 degrees and hold (count to 10) and back to midline, hold (count to 10) and slowly lower to the pad. Do five times to tune up your abdominal and thigh muscles. Increase by five lifts every 3-6 months.

* * * * *

After the Bench Press Lifting or the Barbell Lifting, proceed with the Back, Shoulder, Arm, Abdominal, Hip, and Leg Strengthening Program using your foam pad.

Do push-ups on your foam pad six days a week

OK to do them from the knees with fingers spread. Do five push-ups and increase by five every 3-6 months as tolerated. After your ability to do 25 to 50 from your knees, then progress to doing five pushups from your toes and your fingers to condition and strengthen all the muscle of your fingers, hands, shoulders, back, hips, thighs, knees, ankles and feet. Do 5 push-ups daily from your toes and fingers and increase by 5 every 3-6 months. (If you're unable to progress to the full toes to fingers pushups, continue with the knee to finger pushups.) These are your workout muscle strengthening exercises and there are no upper limits except yours.

Do sit-ups on your foam pad six days a week

Bring your upper body from the lying-on-back position with your hands extended. Raise your back to a full sitting position. With your arms outstretched use your fingers to touch the opposite toes, relax slightly and proceed forward until the other fingers of the opposite hand reach your toes. Do five sit-ups daily. Progress by adding five every 3-6 months as tolerated. These are your workout muscle strengthening exercises and there are no upper limits except yours.

* * * * *

PART III –THE BRAIN

CHAPTER 13

BALANCE COORDINATION AND CONTROL TRAINING

Neurologic Function—Cranial Nerves—Balance Control

　*Balance Coordination and Control Training
　*Stand with feet together: Eyes Open/Closed
　*Stand on One Leg: Eyes Open/Closed
　*Touch object: Close eyes: touch nose, return to object
　*Tandem Walking (Heal to Toe)
　*Touch/Feeling Identifying Objects
　*Vision—Eye training for field of vision, Distance/Nearness Training (ciliary lens muscles exercises)
　*To improve vision to drive without glasses. (20/40 Visual Acuity)

Overview

The neurologic examination as done by your physician includes checking the cranial nerves, a motor and sensory exam, checking the reflexes in each set of muscles, and evaluating balance and coordination. Most physicians now also screen for memory and cognition which will be reviewed in the next chapter.

The motor exam is completed with the ortho exam above. If a set of muscles are weak on one side of the body, or in one extremity, additional evaluation should be obtained from your physician. Generalized weakness may be due to deconditioning. Therefore, you need the strengthening exercises found in this handbook.

The sensory exam is checking the sensation of the skin in all parts of the body. If there is no feeling in one extremity, or one side of the body, it also requires further evaluation and treatment by your physician.

If you note an absence of feeling in your feet and hands, this may be a sign of neuropathy and needs further evaluation by your physician to determine its cause. If there is diabetes in your family, it is likely due to early unsuspected diabetes, which otherwise has few symptoms. Low blood sugar causes symptoms, but moderately high blood sugar does not. That is why a blood glucose test kit is necessary. Kits are readily available OTC and one can check glucose without the expense of a doctor or hospital visit. I checked mine for ten years before my sugars became significantly positive. If that information had been in my medical record, I would have been uninsurable. When one insurance company records diabetes, all insurance companies become aware of it and you become uninsurable except for very high premiums.

With neuropathy, one will have a loss of balance. Dr. Andrew Weil, in his Self-Healing Newsletter recommends balance exercises. As we get older and less active, our balance mechanisms get sluggish because we sit much of the time. Hence, getting active, will improve our balance. All upright activity from walking, jogging, and sports will stimulate balance control. We can test our balance while on our daily walks by making heel-to-toe motions, which helps measure our duration of balance. We can also practice standing with our legs together. If you maintain your balance, proceed with legs together with eyes closed. Be sure to be near a table, hand rail or furniture should you start to fall. If you're successful in this, then try to stand on one foot with eyes open. If successful, close your eyes be sure to be near a table, hand rail or furniture should you start to fall. Doing these exercises daily will help increase your ability to maintain your equilibrium, including sports which require the upright position. Most sports require active balance control and thus are therapeutic.

For more information, peruse Dr. Weil's Self-Healing Newsletter at http://www.drweilnewsletter.com/

Cranial Nerves

There are twelve pairs of cranial nerves that leave the brain through their own passage ways through the skull. They control the functions of the head and neck.

A list of the twelve cranial nerves, the type of nerve (motor or sensory), what number the nerve is, and the function of the nerve are listed for your reference. These are checked in detail on your yearly physical examination and in detail by neurologists.

We will only highlight some major functions and how to maintain their overall functions. These do not need to be done daily or weekly. Check periodically or when abnormalities are suspected. The first two are obviously easy to check.

I.   Olfactory Nerve: Type: Sensory

Function: Sense of Smell (check as needed)

Can you smell flowers, kitchen spices? If you want to develop your sense of smell, see if you can identify flowers or such things as spices without looking at the labels. One can develop the acuity of your sense of smell by noting the smell of various items and learn to identify them.

II.   Optic Nerve: Type: Sensory

Function: Vision

As we age, our range of vision narrows. Keeping this range as wide as possible is also a safety factor in our daily and somewhat hazardous lives, especially when driving.

Check the field of vision by keeping the eye fixed on a distant object, while moving your finger in front of the eye to check vision in all four quadrants. A missing quadrant indicates a serious brain event has occurred. Your visual field should extend to 135 degrees.

*Cranial Nerves III, IV, and VI control the extraocular muscles of the eye. Since the eye moves in all directions, check upward and downward gaze, right and left gaze, and all four oblique gazes.

III. Oculomotor Nerve: Type: Motor

Function: Raise eyelids, move eyes, regulate the size of pupils, focus of lenses

Check accommodation-pupil size as distance changes.

It supplies four extraocular muscles in the eye and the upper eyelids. It controls the muscles that allow for visual tracking and fixation by the eye. Visual tracking is the ability to follow an object as it moves across the field of vision. Fixation is the ability to focus on a stationary object.

IV. Trochlear Nerve: Type: Motor

Function: Eye movements, proprioception (position)

It has the longest pathway and is the smallest nerve to service the eye. It processes brain signals to move the eyes up and down, and outwards. Double vision, otherwise known as diplopia, results from problems with either the muscle or the nerve.

V. Trigeminal Nerve:

Type: Mixed (Motor and sensory)

Function: Primarily responsible for transmitting sensations from the head and face to the brain: the mouth, teeth, face, nasal cavity, chewing movements, and masseter jaw biting, muscle sense.

VI. Abducens Nerve:

Type: Motor

Function: Produce movements of the eyes-lateral gaze

Check to see if eye moves to the left and right margins. If the pupil stays looking forward, you may have a sixth nerve palsy. It can be unilateral or bilateral.

VII. Facial Nerve:

Type: Mixed (Motor and sensory)

Function: Facial expressions (smile, frown), secretion of saliva, taste.

IX. Vestibulocochlear Nerve:

Type: Sensory

Two Functions:

Vestibular: Balance or equilibrium sense.

Cochlear: Hearing. Check both ears.

X. Glossopharyngeal Nerve:

Type: Mixed (Motor and sensory)

Function: Taste and other sensations of tongue (glossus), swallowing (deglutition), secretion of saliva, aid in reflex control of blood pressure and respiration.

XI. Vagus Nerve:

Type: Mixed (Motor and sensory)

Function: Transmit impulses to muscles associated with speech, swallowing, the heart, smooth muscles of visceral organs in the thorax, and abdomen. (Vagal reflex slows the heart rate: the Valsalva maneuver.)

XII. Accessory Nerve:

Type: Motor

Function: Turning movements of the head, movements of the shoulder and viscera, voice production. Check by raising both shoulders and rotation of the head.

XIII. Hypoglossal Nerve:

Type: Motor

Function: Tongue movements (force tongue against finger on both cheeks to check muscles on both sides of tongue.)

Balance Control

1. The gaze stabilization system maintains gaze direction of the eyes and visual acuity during activities involving active head and body movements. Gaze stabilization and the vestibulo-ocular reflex (VOR) systems are often viewed as synonymous, even though the VOR is only one component of gaze stabilization.

2. The postural stabilization system keeps the body in balance while an individual is standing and actively moves about in daily life.

The gaze and postural stability systems are distinct because they rely on information from different senses, motor reactions of different parts of the body, and are mediated by different brain pathways. The two systems are, however, interdependent because gaze stability is not possible unless the body on which the head and eyes ride is also stable and because accurate vision is a critical sensory input to postural control, which is dependent on gaze stability.

Balance exercises therefore, must involve balance while standing with our eyes open as well as closed. With our eyes open we can constantly check and correct balance problems visually. If this is normal, then doing the same test with eyes closed will check if our postural stabilization is effective. If we lose our balance with eyes closed, we need practice to stabilize our balance mechanism. As we get older and more sedentary, this system is used less, and we lose our balance more easily. So, to reactivate the postural stabilization system, we check our ability to stand with eyes closed. We do a partial stimulation every time we stand on one leg to put on our trousers. We can increase this stimulation by delaying the second leg as long as we can maintain our balance.

If you're unsteady, check the length of time you can stand. Then proceed to stand on one foot and measure the amount of time you can maintain balance. Do the same with the other foot. Dr. Weil maintains that you can improve your balance by doing this daily. By measuring the seconds or minutes each day, one should see improvement.

Another good exercise is heel-to-toe walking on a straight line. Be sure to do this next to a stable or fixed object such as a counter so you can stabilize yourself if you become wobbly. If you can do this with your eyes open practice with your eyes closed.

Also place your finger on an object such as a knob on a chair. Then close your eyes and move the finger to your nose and back to the chair. Do this also by moving the finger to your ear and back to the chair. If your position sense is in good order, you can find any part of your body with your eyes closed. You should be able to re-find any part of another object by returning to your body and then the other object. In the examination room, the doctor holds your finger, has you close your eyes, and asks you to go to your nose and then return to his finger to check your position sense.

* * * * *

To test for the cranial nerves, go to: http://www.ivyroses.com/HumanBody/Nerves/Cranial-Nerves.php

* * * * *

Doctor/Patient anecdote:

I was examining a doctor and noted that he was a bit unsteady for the age of 40. When I did the finger to nose test, he missed his nose by 4 inches and missed the return to my outstretched finger by six inches. "Do you sometimes miss your mouth when you eat?" "Yes, all the time. I just thought that I was getting sloppy."

He had diabetic neuropathy and didn't know he had diabetes.

A physician should obtain consultation when the abnormality is so gross.

* * * * *

You can further evaluate your sense of touch or feeling by closing your eyes while someone puts an object, such as a ball, fruit, or tool in your hand. Then try to identify the object by touch and feel.

For more detailed information concerning balance, go to http://balanceandmobility.com/for-clinicians/the-balance-control-system/

For balance improvement exercises, also see http://www.thebalancemanual.com/?device=c&gclid=EAIaIQo bChMIjJy0nsie1wIVD0R-Ch2naAT6EAAYASAAEgI3afD_BwE

* * * * *

Anecdote:

In medical school, a classmate decided he wanted to be an ophthalmologist when he entered practice. He also wanted to have perfect vision. He had a meter ruler with a track mounted dot which he could move back and forth to exercise the muscles of his lenses. One can watch the pupillary reflex by doing this. He would begin by looking far away and then focusing on intermediate objects moving to the dot at the end of his meter stick. Next he would move that dot to his nose keeping his focus on it until his eyes crossed.

You can do the same exercise for the lenses without any gadgetry by looking far away and gradually bringing your gaze to objects closer. Then you can use your finger bringing your gaze in a few inches from your nose until your eyes cross. This exercises the ciliary muscles around the lens that changes the convexity of the lens for near and far vision. This helps keep the lens soft and functioning. My classmate met his goal of becoming an ophthalmologist with essentially perfect vision that didn't require corrective glasses.

This is a good eye exercise you can do frequently during the course of the day even while doing your aerobics.

For detail cranial nerve exam and discussion, go to . . . http://www.neuroexam.com/neuroexam/content19.html
For further discussion of the cranial nerves, go to . . . https://en.wikipedia.org/wiki/Cranial_nerves

CHAPTER 14

MEMORY—COGNITION IMPROVEMENT EXERCISES

The Brain

"The Brain is a terrible thing to waste"- by Russell Blaylock, MD. He is the author of several popular books on nutrition and wellness and is medical editor of the Newsmax monthly newsletter /Blaylock Wellness Report/. He is a member of the international board of the World Natural Health Organization and serves on the editorial staff of the /Journal of the American Nutraceutical Association/.

As a neurosurgeon for 25 years, Dr. Blaylock has peeked inside the brains of thousands of people. Time and time again he's seen someone's miraculous brain turn from friend to foe.

He's observed over 60% of people middle-aged and older suffer some degree of memory impairment.

And according to the National Institute on Aging, memory problems are one of the first warning signs of cognitive loss, which involves mental slowing and declining intellect. As cognitive loss takes hold, the lights are still on, but they grow dimmer with time.

Some years back, Dr. Blaylock turned his focus from conventional medicine and neurosurgery to nutrition and natural health. He saw that far too many physicians were not addressing the underlying causes for health issues.

Instead, he observed most mainstream doctors relying too heavily on methods which only mask symptoms. He believed you deserve better than that. See references in Bibliography

You Have a Living 'Forest' of Nerve Cells in Your Brain

The average brain contains about 100 billion nerve cells or neurons. These neurons branch out and connect at about one trillion points. This is such a vast and dense network of connections, scientists call it a "neuron forest."

Your neurons communicate with each other through connecting points known as synapses.

The signals that form your memories and thoughts move across your neurons as minute electric charges. When these charges reach a synapse, they trigger the release of chemicals called neurotransmitters. These chemical messengers travel across the synapse, carrying signals to other nerve cells in progression.

Unfortunately, with increasing age, the brain undergoes a lot of changes that affect these processes:

* Certain areas of the brain will shrink, including the hippocampus and the prefrontal cortex. These are particularly important parts of the brain when it comes to memory, learning, and other complex mental activities.

* Neurons also shrink. The connections between the neurons deteriorate and become less extensive, and the level of neurotransmitters may decrease.

* The aging brain undergoes a gradual reduction in blood flow.

* Aging accelerates the process of inflammation in the brain as well as the entire body.

* Free radicals in the brain and body accumulate at a faster rate with age.

* Free radicals are highly reactive molecules that can damage neurons and other body cells.

These are just a few reasons why maintaining the function of your nerve cells, neurotransmitters, and your brain's "forest" is crucial to your memory and your ability to think — particularly as you grow older.

Which of These 5 Common Brain Aging & Memory Concerns Do You Have?

* Forgetting where you put your car keys or glasses

* Noticing problems finding the right word when speaking

* Forgetting appointments — or the names of people you just met

* Feeling "scatterbrained" and unable to concentrate or focus on tasks

* A foggy brain feeling that keeps you from thinking clearly

Fortunately, there are some simple ways to help support your memory and brain health as the years pass. The strategies recommended by Dr. Blaylock can be found on his website under: 7 Tips to Keep Your Mental Edge as You Grow Older.

Dr. Blaylock spent years studying the latest findings on nutrition and brain health. To that end, he found that five nutrients play an important role in supporting optimal brain function.

To read more, please go to: http://www.blaylockreport.com/ or subscribe to the Wellness Report wherein he shares some crucial information to help you keep your mental edge — naturally.

Memory & Cognition

Cognition is a term referring to the mental processes involved in gaining knowledge and comprehension. These processes include thinking, knowing, remembering, judging and problem-solving. These are higher-level functions of the brain and encompass language, imagination, perception, and planning.

Memory is the process of maintaining information over time." (Matlin, 2005)

Memory is the means by which we draw on our past experiences in order to use this information in the present.' (Sternberg, 1999)

Memory is the term given to the structures and processes involved in the storage and subsequent retrieval of information.

Memory is essential to all our lives. Without a memory of the past we cannot operate in the present or think about the future. We would not be able to remember what we did yesterday, what we have done today or what we plan to do tomorrow. Without memory we could not learn anything.

Memory is involved in processing vast amounts of information. This information takes many different forms, e.g.

images, sounds or meaning. There has been a significant amount of research regarding the differences between Short Term Memory (STM) and Long Term Memory (LTM).

For psychologists the term memory covers three important aspects of information processing:

Encoding:

1. Visual (picture)

2. Acoustic (sound)

3. Semantic (meaning)

For example, how do you remember a telephone number you have looked up in the phone book? If you can see it then you are using visual coding, but if you are repeating it to yourself you are using acoustic coding (by sound). Evidence suggests that acoustic coding is the principle coding system in short term memory (STM).

The principle encoding system in long term memory (LTM) appears to be semantic coding (by meaning).

However, information in LTM can also be coded both visually and acoustically.

Most adults can store between five and nine items in their short-term memory.

This is the basis for one of the screening tests for Alzheimer disease. Physicians will frequently give the patient five items to memorize at the beginning of a visit. They are asked to form a sentence with each of the items. At the end of the examination, the physician asks the patient to recite them. If the patient remembers four out of five, their memory is considered normal.

Some patients come in with a chief complaint of feeling they have Alzheimer's. Here the screenings tests are not adequate and neurologic consultation is required which will include a more complete neurologic, mental status and MRI of the brain exam. I have never had a patient return from the neurologist with a diagnosis of Alzheimer's. But I know that my screening tests would never satisfy a patient who is in dread of the disease. Hence, a neurology referral is required to allay the patient's concerns.

Personal Anecdote:

When I applied for disability insurance, the company sent out an RN to do the exam because I was approaching 60. She gave me ten items asking me to form a sentence with each. An hour later at the end of the exam she asked me to name the ten items. I got six, and she looked concerned. Then I remembered the 7th. So, she passed me as not being at risk for Alzheimer's. Whew!

Medical Anecdote

We have all observed medical students, interns, residents, and fellows who carry a small ring binder in their white coats. These have always been referred to as a doctor's "peripheral brain." As new facts, findings, or diseases were studied, they were entered on to the pages of the peripheral brain. We visualized the facts (Visual encoding); we repeated them as we entered the facts (Acoustic encoding) and then entered a few additional words so we could recall the meaning (Semantic encoding). Thus, the new medical findings could always be accessed to recollect memories of learning. Thus, we stimulated visual, acoustic and semantic encoding.

Most doctors put aside these on entering practice because they were a negative observation for their patients.

Recently as these physicians have aged, I've notice that more of them have returned to keeping a peripheral brain or a diary/journal. This has improved their memory as they enter items in their peripheral brain, visualize them, whisper them out loud, and enter a word or two to help recall their meaning. Thus, the peripheral brain is returning as an adjunct to memory as memory fades.

I've recently returned to this practice as I've noted many of my colleagues have done so also. When I see them at the medical conferences, they have their diary/journal (peripheral brain) with them. Now they also record their personal medical information such as their BP, Glucose levels, cholesterol levels, (so they speak knowledgeably with their own doctors on the next visit). They also record the names of colleagues they speak with at the conference as well as some new concepts from the faculty presenters. This may be an appropriate hedge to diminishing memory.

I personally have seen an improvement in my memory and recollection of facts by having this year long journal with me at all times. The physician seated next to me stated he had 40 volumes of his diary which he felt were very helpful in recall. I think we can now recommend this as an appropriate adjunct for the aging brain.

Keep exercising your BRAIN through visual, acoustical and semantic channels. These can be enhanced with a small diary or journal to record visual and semantic channels of memory retention.

The BRAIN controls your body.

Keep it active.

It's a terrible thing to waste.

EPILOGUE

A restaurant unashamed of its high-calorie, unhealthy menu

http://www.medicalnewstoday.com/articles/218313.php?utm_source=TrendMD&utm_medium=cpc&utm_campaign=Medical_News_Today_TrendMD_0

By Christian Nordqvist, 5 March 2011

Blair River, 6ft 8inches tall, spokesman for the Heart Attack Grill, died at age 29 from what appeared to be a complication of flu - pneumonia. The 575-pound man's job was to promote a restaurant unashamed of its high-calorie, unhealthy menu.

At Chandler's Heart Attack Grill, staff walk around in nurse's uniforms and the owner, John Basso, has a doctor's white coat - however, the menu is definitely not for those interested in good health or looking after their figure.

The restaurant has meals in excess of 8,000 calories. An active 200lbs man who is 6ft 2ins tall does not require more than 2,000 calories per day. This man at 6ft 8in would not require more than 2,500 calories per day. Consuming 8,000 in just one sitting, plus whatever else that person might eat during their other meals would most definitely result in excessive weight gain. The menu features milkshakes, French fries cooked in pig lard and giant hamburgers.

A large sign warns "Caution. This establishment is bad for your health."

Basso and several regular clients say that it is all a question of choice, nobody is making anyone eat there, it is a personal decision.

Having River, a giant of a man, as the restaurant's spokesman was part of a humorous glorification of obesity.

Basso says River's death is no laughing matter. "You couldn't have found a better person", he said. He added that those who knew him are crying their eyes out.

Even if River had been skinny he would still have been given the job, according to Basso.

FOOD GLUTONY HAS NO LIMITS.

APPENDIX ONE

Diets with Biographies for Optional Further Reading

From Peanuts: You can eat all you want, but you can't swallow. After Snoopy throws the dog dish at Charlie Brown, he awakens from his concussion stating, "It's no fun being a waiter if you can't joke with the customers!"

Obesity is not a laughing matter for the obese patients. You better not try to joke with them. Sometimes it's hard to be serious with them or even bring up the subject of their weight. But then, it is no wonder that people get confused reading diet books. The messages indeed are confusing. I hope this has been helpful. Thank you to all the publishers for sending me copies of their books.

Diets - Some of them work. Some of them don't.

And some are just plain dangerous. Extreme diet fads have become a part of our culture. Hundreds are found on the various websites.

The following are the recommended diets and food plans. You may want to review the ones I did as Editor of Sacramento Medicine at www.DelMeyer.net.

* * * * *

PORTION SAVVY, THE 30-DAY SMART PLAN FOR EATING WELL

BY CARRIE LATT WIATT

Very informative; Ms. Wiatt posts an entire chapter on her website which gives the fundaments of her Portion Savvy program which is excellent. The 30-day Smart Plan for Eating Well (Pocket Books, $24) was written by Carrie Latt Wiatt, who has a Master's Degree in nutrition. She is Hollywood's favorite nutritionist and feels that in 30 days she can inspire you to a healthier and happier body. She says her PS men and women don't diet–they manage food wisely. She recognizes the struggles that are peculiar to our country since she has an international clientele. People moving here from other countries are amazed at the portions "they serve you here." She wonders if the custom officials should warn people about the overfeeding of America. No country in the world eats as much as we do or struggles with weight problems and nutritional diseases as we do. Recognizing that we are conditioned to over eat in America, she offers guidelines on changing our habits in a very readable and relatable format. Read the first chapter online.

* * * * *

THE ZONE DIET
BY BARRY SEARS, PHD

This is a very comprehensive nutritional program, which is easily put into action. After a discussion of the ill effects of hyperinsulinism, he presents a system of balanced eating so one always remains "in the zone." He sees no need to buy exercise equipment or join a gym or pay to exercise. Read the first three chapters and then replace the book in your book case. Let's keep matters simple.

* * * * *

EATING WELL FOR OPTIMUM HEALTH
BY ANDREW WEIL, MD

This is a very comprehensive guide to food, diet, and nutrition. As a clinical professor of medicine at the University of Arizona, and director of the Program in Integrative Medicine, he speaks with authority and writes in textbook fashion. However, it is very readable.

* * * * *

THE PRITIKIN DIET PROGRAM
BY NATHAN PRITIKIN

This is scientifically accurate, but severe. The Pritikin Diet Programs of Nathan Pritikin have been continued by his son Robert, director of the Pritikin Longevity Center. The current volume, The New Pritikin Program by Robert Pritikin (Pocket Books, $7) is friendlier and more in tune with a lifetime commitment. The results of the first 893 people that participated in the 26-day Pritikin Longevity Center program was published in 1974 and was evaluated by the Department of Biostatistics and Epidemiology at Loma Linda University. The results indicated that 83% of hypertensive people lowered their blood pressure to normal and left the program drug-free; 50% of adult-onset diabetics on insulin left the program free of insulin; 90% of diabetics on oral drugs left free of drugs; 62% of drug-taking angina patients left the center drug free; cholesterol and triglycerides were each lowered an average of 25%; overweight people lost an average of 13 pounds; of the 64 people who were recommended for bypass surgery, 80 % of them had not undergone surgery even five years later. Read my review at:

http://www.delmeyer.net/MedicalLiterature/bookshelf/Diets.htm

* * * * *

DIETS DON'T WORK
BY BOB SCHWARTZ, PHD

This book is very insightful, humorous, informative and popular. It is now in its third edition. Read the first chapter online.

* * * * *

DIETS STILL DON'T WORK
BY BOB SCHWARTZ, PHD

http://www.delmeyer.net/MedicalLiterature/bookshelf/Diets.htm#Portion%20Savvy,%20The%2030-

LIVE WELL

APPENDIX TWO

Foods That Spike Blood Sugar and should be avoided

1. Sugary foods such as: sodas, cake, candy, and sweets

   Eat fruits like berries, apples, pears and oranges in small amounts.

2. Fruit juices:

   Juice has concentrated sugars, as do most sweet fruits. Go to plain or flavored seltzer with a spritz of lemon or lime.

3. Dried fruit:

   Although it contains fiber and nutrients, the dehydration process causes fruits natural juices to get super concentrated.

   Skip dried fruits and go to fresh fruits: grapefruit, strawberries, cantaloupe, peaches, but in small amounts.

4. White rice, bread, flour, refined starches:

   These DIGEST like sugar. "White Carbs" sharply raise glucose levels. Whole grains such as brown or wild rice, barley, oatmeal, high fiber cereals and whole grain breads raise blood glucose less than refined grains, but they still are carbohydrates, so be cautious, and check your blood glucose after eating them.

5. Full fat dairy products:

   Some studies indicate not only do saturated fats raise your "bad" cholesterol, but saturated fats may worsen insulin resistance.

   Do your best to avoid dairy products made with whole milk such as cream, full fat yogurt, ice cream, cream cheese, and other full fat cheeses. One percent milk has three fourths of the fat removed. Look for reduced fat or fat free dairy products instead.

6. Fatty cuts of meat:

   These are high in saturated fats, just like whole milk dairy products. It can put people with diabetes at an even greater risk for heart disease than the average person. Choose lean proteins including skinless chicken and turkey, fish and shell fish, pork tenderloin and lean beef.

7. Packaged snacks and baked goods:

Aside from all the sugar, white flour, sodium and the preservatives they contain packaged snacks and baked goods like chips, doughnuts and snack cakes often have trans fats.

Trans fats increase your "bad" cholesterol (LDL) and lower your "good" cholesterol (HDL) and can raise your risk for heart disease.

8. For diabetics, no amount of trans fats is deemed safe since they are dangerous for causing heart disease.

Avoid partially hydrogenated oils, a major source of trans fats. Seek out healthy fats in salmon and other fish as well as nuts, seeds, avocado, olive and canola oil.

9. Fried foods:

You may have a weakness for French Fries, fried chicken, potato chips and the like, but kicking this craving is good for your long-term health. Fried foods typically soak up tons of oil (lots of extra calories) and many are coated with breading first, jacking up the numbers even more. To add insult to injury, some foods are deep fried in hydrogenated oils which are laden with unhealthy trans fats.

10. Alcohol:

Alcohol can interfere with blood sugar levels. If you do drink, keep it in "moderation." Moderation is generally defined as no more than one serving a day for women and two for men. A typical serving is measured as 5 ounces of wine, 12 ounces of beer, or 1-½ ounces of liquor.

11. The Glycemic Index:

This index ranks food on a scale from 0 to 100; the closer to 100, the higher the glycemic index. Glucose, a unit of carbohydrate broken down into its simplest form, has a glycemic index of 100. Foods below 55 have a low glycemic index, foods between 56 and 69 have a medium glycemic index and foods above 70 have a high glycemic index. To determine a food's glycemic index, volunteers eat 50 grams of carbohydrate. Participants' blood sugar levels are measured for the next two hours and compared to the changes in their blood sugar levels after eating 50 grams of glucose, which is the reference food of the glycemic index.

APPENDIX THREE

FOODS TO EAT IF YOU HAVE TYPE 2 DIABETES

1. Beans: Black, White, Navy, Lima, Pinto, Soy, Garbanzo and Kidney

Good, high quality carbohydrates, lean protein, and soluble fiber that not only helps to stabilize blood sugar levels but keeps hunger in check (virtually fat free).

2. Oatmeal:

Studies have shown that eating a diet rich in whole grains and high fiber may reduce the risk of diabetes between 35% and 42%. Oatmeal is an excellent source of both.

3. Fish: An excellent source of protein

Catfish, cod, tilapia are good. Prepare healthfully by baking, grilling, or roasting.

4. Non-Fat Yogurt:

Fat free yogurt contains both high quality carbs and protein making it an excellent food for slowing or preventing an unhealthy rise in blood sugar. Studies also show that a diet high in calcium from yogurt and other calcium rich foods is associated with a reduced risk of type 2 diabetes. Be sure to stick to non-fat brands. Non-fat Greek Yogurt is excellent.

5. Almonds:

Unsalted almonds provide a healthy low carb mix of monounsaturated fats plus magnesium which is believed to be instrumental in carbohydrate metabolism. A Harvard study found that high daily magnesium intake reduced the risk of developing diabetes by 33%. Therefore, including more magnesium rich foods like almonds, pumpkin seeds, spinach, and Swiss chard in your diet is a smart move.

6. Non-Starchy Vegetables:

Chock full of vitamins, minerals and fiber, non-starchy vegetables such as broccoli, spinach, mushrooms, and peppers are an ideal source of high quality carbohydrates. They have a low impact on blood sugar. And it's okay to eat as much as you like.

7. Wild Salmon:

Wild salmon or sardines are not only rich in heart healthy Omega-3's but also contain a healthy fat and protein combination that slows the body's absorption of carbs keeping blood sugars on an even keel.

8. Egg Whites:

Rich in high quality lean protein and low in carbs, egg whites are another healthy choice for controlling or preventing Type-2 diabetes. One large egg white contains about 16 calories and 4 grams of high quality filling protein making egg whites a perfect food for blood sugar control, not to mention weight loss.

9. Avocado:

Avocado is high in monounsaturated fats which are generally considered among the healthiest of fats. Researchers have found that a diet high in monounsaturated fats and low in low quality carbs may improve insulin sensitivity. Add avocado to your sandwiches instead of mayo.

APPENDIX FOUR

Fat Facts:

Saturated fats come mostly from animal products although some plant foods like coconut, cacao, and palm oil contain it also. It elevates levels of low-density lipoproteins (LDL) cholesterol, which increases cardiovascular disease. This is also found in many snacks and non-dairy food such as coffee creamers, whipped toppings.

Monounsaturated fats, such as avocados, nuts, olive oil, helps lower LDL and rise high density lipoprotein (HDL) the good cholesterol.

Polyunsaturated fats, as found in fish, flaxseed, soybean oil, lowers LDL

Trans fats, a fat that has been changed by a process called hydrogenation. It raises the LDLs and lowers the HDLs and thus increases heart and vascular disease risks. This process increases the shelf life of fats and makes the fat more solid at room temperatures, as found in margarine, shortening, commercial baked goods. It makes crackers crispier and pie crusts flakier.

* * * * *

Here are 10 high-fat foods that are incredibly healthy and nutritious.

https://www.healthline.com/nutrition/10-super-healthy-high-fat-foods#section1

Ever since fat was demonized, people started eating more sugar, refined carbs and processed foods instead. As a result, the entire world has become fatter and sicker.

However, times are changing. Studies now show that fat, including saturated fat, isn't the devil it was made out to be. All sorts of healthy foods that happen to contain fat have now returned to the "superfood" scene.

105

Here are 10 high-fat foods that are incredibly healthy and nutritious.

- Avocados
- Cheese
- Dark Chocolate
- Whole Eggs
- Fatty Fish
- Nuts
- Chia Seeds
- Extra Virgin Olive Oil
- Coconuts and Coconut Oil
- Yogurt

However, use in small amounts.

APPENDIX FIVE

Top 10 Foods Highest in Sodium By Daisy Whitbread, MScN

https://www.healthaliciousness.com/articles/what-foods-high-sodium.php

Foods high in Sodium (Salt)

Sodium is an essential nutrient required by the body for maintaining proper blood pressure and for providing channels of nerve signaling. Deficiency of sodium is rare but can occur in people after excessive vomiting or diarrhea, in athletes who consume excessive amounts of water, or in people who regularly fast on juice and water. Over-consumption of sodium is far more common and can lead to high blood pressure which in turn leads to an increased risk of heart attack and stroke. The current percent daily value (%DV) for sodium is 2400mg, however, the American Heart Association recommends that people with high blood pressure eat less than 1500mg per day, or less than 3/4 of a table spoon of salt. Since sodium is required by all life to exist, it is naturally found in all foods and rarely does salt ever need to be added. Foods high in sodium include table salt, sauces, salad dressings, cured meats, bacon, pickles, bullion, instant soup, roasted salted nuts, snacks, fast foods, and canned foods.

The following is a list of high sodium foods; for more, see the extended lists of high sodium foods by nutrient density, list of high sodium foods to boost sodium levels, and the list of high sodium foods to avoid.

#1: Table Salt, Baking Soda & Baking Powder (Table Salt)

I. Sodium 100g	Per tablespoon (18g)	Per teaspoon (6g)
38758mg (1615% DV)	6976mg (291% DV)	2325mg (97% DV)

Baking Soda & Baking Powder Are Also High in Sodium (%DV per teaspoon). Baking Soda (57%) and Baking Powder (22%). Click to see complete nutrition facts.

#2: Sauces & Salad Dressings (Soy Sauce)

Sodium 100g	Per tablespoon (18g)	Per teaspoon (6g)
6820mg (284% DV)	1228mg (51% DV)	409mg (17% DV)

Other Sauces and Dressings High in Sodium (%DV per tablespoon): Fish Sauce (59%), Teriyaki (29%), Oyster Sauce (21%), Hot Pepper Sauce & Reduced-Salt Soy Sauce (18%), Steak Sauce (12%), Reduced-Fat Salad Dressing (11%), Barbeque Sauce, Worcestershire Sauce & Hamburger Relish (7%). Click to see complete nutrition facts.

#3: Cured Meat & Fish (Bacon, Cooked)

Sodium 100g	Per ounce (28g)	Per slice (8g)
2193mg(91% DV)	614mg (25% DV)	175mg (7% DV)

Other Cured Meat & Fish High in Sodium (%DV per ounce): Salt Cod (82%), Salted Mackerel (52%), Canned Anchovy (43%), Dried Beef (32%), Turkey Bacon & Salami (27%), Beef Jerky (24%), Smoked Salmon (23%), Italian Salami (22%), Smoked White Fish (12%), and Smoked Herring (11%). Click to see complete nutrition facts.

#4: Cheese (Roquefort)

Sodium 100g	Per package (85g)	Per ounce (28g)
1809mg(75% DV)	1538mg(64% DV)	507mg (21% DV)

Other Cheeses High in Sodium (%DV per ounce): Queso Seco (21%), Romano (17%), Parmesan (16%), Blue Cheese (13%), Feta (11%), Camembert & Gouda (10%). Click to see complete nutrition facts.

#5: Pickles (Cucumber)

Sodium 100g	Per cup (155g)	Per pickle (65g)
1208mg(50% DV)	1872mg(78% DV)	785mg (33% DV)

Other Pickles High in Sodium (%DV per cup): Olives (117%), Pickled Eggplant (95%), Jalapeno Peppers (72%), and Sauerkraut (39%). Click to see complete nutrition facts.

6: Instant Soups (Beef Noodle)

Sodium 100g	Per ounce (28g)	Per packet (9g)
8408mg (350% DV)	2354mg (98% DV)	757mg (32% DV)

Other Instant Soups High in Sodium (%DV per packet): Onion (131%), Chicken Noodle (112%), Tomato & Vegetable (109%), 1 Bullion (Stock) Cube (50% DV), and Cream of Vegetable Soup (37%). Click to see complete nutrition facts.

#7: Roasted and Salted Nuts & Seeds (Pumpkin Seeds)

Sodium 100g	Per cup (64g)	Per ounce (28g)
2541mg (106% DV)	1626mg (68% DV)	711mg (30% DV)

Other Roasted and Salted Nuts and Seeds High in Sodium (%DV per ounce): Almonds (8%), Cashew Nuts and Sunflower Seeds (7%), and Pistachio Nuts (5%). Click to see complete nutrition facts.

#8: Snacks (Pretzels)

Sodium 100g	Per 10 twists (60g)	Per ounce (28g)
1715mg (71% DV)	1029mg (43% DV)	480mg (20% DV)

Other Snacks High in Sodium (%DV per ounce): Sesame Sticks (17%), Reduced-Fat Tortilla Chips (12%), Salted Popcorn, Soy Chips and Pita Chips (10%), and Salted Peanuts (9%). Click to see complete nutrition facts.

#9: Fast Foods (Egg & Ham Biscuit)

Sodium 100g	Per biscuit (182g)	Per 3oz (85g)
1093mg (46% DV)	1989mg (83% DV)	929mg (39% DV)

Other Fast Foods High in Sodium (%DV per piece, serving or slice): Beef & Cheese Enchilada (55%), Beef, Chili & Cheese Burrito (44%), Applebee's French Fries (42%), Wendy's Jr. Hamburger with Cheese (35%), Thin Crust Pepperoni Pizza (29%), and Hush Puppies (10%). Click to see complete nutrition facts.

#10: Canned Vegetables (Sweet Peppers)

Sodium 100g	Per cup (140g)	Per 1/2 cup (70g)
1369mg (57% DV)	1917mg (80% DV)	956mg (40% DV)

Other Canned Vegetables High in Sodium (%DV per cup): Jalapeno Peppers (72%), Tomato Sauce (54%), Snap Beans (36%), Zucchini (35%), Spinach (29%), Asparagus and Mushrooms (28%), Peas, Onions & Sweetcorn (22%), Sun Dried Tomatoes (12%). Click to see complete nutrition facts.

For excellent references on numerous food lists, go to the website by Daisy Whitbread, MScH:

https://www.healthaliciousness.com/

BIBLIOGRAPHY

Centers for Disease Control:
Explore additional information:
https://www.cdc.gov/physicalactivity/basics/pa-health/index.htm#LiveLonger

Bob Schwartz, PhD:
DIETS DON'T WORK 3rd ED Paperback – February 25, 2015
https://www.amazon.com/DIETS-DONT-WORK-3RD-ED/dp/0942540166
http://www.delmeyer.net/MedicalLiterature/bookshelf/bkrev_D ietsDon'tWork.htm

Carrie Latt Wiatt:
Further reading on -Portion Control Diet Plan: Read an entire chapter on Carrie Latt's Amazon Website:
https://www.amazon.com/gp/product/0671024175#reader_067 1024175
http://www.delmeyer.net/MedicalLiterature/bookshelf/Diets.ht m#Portion%20Savvy,%20The%2030-

Further reading: Purdue Diet: Diet-Related Diseases:
http://www.four-h.purdue.edu/foods/Diet-Related%20Diseases.htm

Nathan Pritikin:
The Lost Lectures from Nathan Pritikin
Listen to his lectures:
https://www.drmcdougall.com/health/education/podcast/nathan -pritikin/
Autopsy of Pritikin
http://articles.latimes.com/1985-07-04/news/vw-9280_1_nathan-pritikin

Mayo Clinic Diet Plans

https://www.mayoclinic.org/healthy-lifestyle/weight-loss/in-depth/weight-loss/art-20048466?pg=2

Antioxidants

https://w3.mindhealthreport.com/Health/MHR/Offers/MHR-Younger-Brain-OP?dkt_nbr=ujmjf5kq

UCSF Guidelines for a Low Sodium Diet

https://www.ucsfhealth.org/education/guidelines_for_a_low_sodium_diet/

Daisy Whitbread, MScN

https://www.healthaliciousness.com/

Rachel Bachman:

Gyms Ditch Machines to Make Space for Free Weights
As boutique-style workouts become the norm, the ranks of cardio and weight machines are thinning.

Russell Blaylock, MD:

A Brain Is a Terrible Thing to Waste;
https://www.newsmax.com/health/

AFTERWORD—SUMMARY

You now have the outline for lifelong healthy living.
Keep this booklet handy for quick and frequent reference.
Download a personal copy (available after your purchase)
Order a DVD of the Exercise Program (pending)
Order a CD of the Book (pending)

www.ingramcontent.com/pod-product-compliance
Lightning Source LLC
Chambersburg PA
CBHW031214270326
41931CB00006B/560